The Low-FODMAP Diet Cookbook for Beginners

Easy and Gut-Friendly Low-FODMAP Recipes for IBS
Relief and Other Digestive Disorders

By Alice Tony

Table of Contents

Introduction

I believe that food does not only satiate our hunger and fuel our daily activities, but it also provides nourishment and well-being to the body. Having said this, the types of food that we eat can either make or break us. Growing up, I suffered from having a sensitive stomach, and it was only later that I realized after becoming a nutritionist that food plays a vital role in our well-being. Moreover, I have also realized that food has healing abilities such that the regular stomach upset that I experienced since childhood can be reverse by knowing which foods to eat and which to avoid.

And so, I started with my quest not only into healthy eating but also finding as much as I can about foods that are bad for people with digestive distress. This is where my journey into the low FODMAP diet began. I have tried different kinds of diets that were supposedly designed for people with a sensitive stomach, but the low FODMAP diet is where I became successful. The low FODMAP diet is all about restricting your intake of fermentable carbohydrates known as FODMAPs. Amazed by its success in relieving my digestive issues, I began my intensive research on this diet until I decided to write this book in the hopes that it may help many people as well.

If you suffer from digestive problems such as irritable bowel syndrome (IBS), bloating, and indigestion, and you want a diet that is friendly to your sensitive gut, then this book is for you. I created this book in the hopes that people may be able to alleviate their digestive problems through the food that they eat. As someone who believes in empirical evidence, this diet is backed by science as this particular diet is the subject of several studies on nutrition. Long before it was turned into a full diet regimen, a low FODMAP diet has been clinically recommended for the management of the symptoms of IBS. But more than people who suffer from problems with digestion, this book is excellent for everyone who wants to follow a healthy and holistic diet.

And so, I want to share everything that I have learned about my research on the low FODMAP diet for you. I understand that the low FODMAP diet is something that you might not have heard of before. Compared with the other types of diet that have been around for quite a while, the low FODMAP diet has been under the radar. And so, I wrote this book to remove any obscurities involving the low FODMAP diet. Thus, with this book, you will be able to learn about the etiology of gut problems and how eating the right kinds of food can help relieve your situation. Moreover, this book will also discuss how you can stick with this diet and enjoy its benefits long term. This book will also feature healthy and easy-to-follow recipes so that you can jumpstart your way to a gut-friendly diet. Enjoy!

The Fodmap Diet: Everything You Need To Know About This Diet

Not all foods are created equally such that while some foods can have healing effects, others can trigger digestive problems, especially among people who suffer from a sensitive digestive tract. This is the reason why it is so crucial for people who have sensitive stomachs to be very careful with the types of foods that they consume. While there are different types of diets that you can follow, if you want to address your stomach issues specifically, then the low FODMAP diet is for you.

Chapter 1: The Etiology of Gut Problems

Before we discuss the low FODMAP diet, you must understand the etiology of gut problems and the digestive system itself. This chapter will cover the

Everything Starts with The Digestive Tract

Everything starts with the digestive system. The digestive system is one of the most extensive and intricate parts of the body as it does not only comprise the stomach and intestines, but it ranges from the mouth down to the rectum. The digestive system is responsible not only for the mechanical and chemical digestion of food, but it is also responsible for the absorption of essential nutrients, metabolism, and removal of wastes from the body. Thus, problems related to digestion can warrant many unwanted symptoms and, if left untreated, can lead to more serious as well as chronic diseases.

So how does digestion work? Think of your digestive system as an efficient conveyor belt. The process of digestion begins at the mouth where food particles are broken down via mechanical digestion using the teeth and part chemical digestion through the saliva. Once you have chewed the food, it moves into the food pipe called esophagus until it reaches the stomach. From the stomach, the food is further broken down using the stomach acid to breakdown protein and release the nutrients for easy absorption.

Moreover, the food also comes into contact with the enzymes found in the pancreas that can further break the food as well as bile that breaks down lipids. It then travels to the small intestines where the microvilli absorb the nutrients on the internal surface of the intestines. This time, the food particles already become a bolus and are then sent to the large intestines – the last stop of the digestive process – where it is passed out as poo from the rectal orifice.

How Food Triggers Digestive Problems

The food that you eat can trigger digestive problems, especially if you have a sensitive gut in the first place. When you regularly suffer from gut problems, and your doctor cannot find any underlying reason for your problem, then what you have is a functional gastrointestinal disorder. How food triggers digestive problems can vary from one individual to another.

For instance, a person who is highly lactose intolerant does lack the enzyme lactase that breaks down milk and dairy products. But even if you have normal biochemistry, there are really certain types of foods that can add stress to the digestive system.

Consumption of fatty or fried foods can stimulate the contractions in the digestive tract, which results in the speeding up of the digestion, causing diarrhea or slowing down the emptying of the stomach causing constipation. If you suffer from irritable bowel syndrome, it can help if you create a food diary and list down certain foods that can trigger your condition.

Types of Digestive Problems That Can Be Addressed by Low FODMAP Diet

There are so many types of digestion problems that can be addressed by eating the right kinds of food. However, it is crucial to take note that the FODMAP diet can address not all types of digestion problems. Specifically, this particular diet can address the following:

- **Irritable Bowel Syndrome:** Irritable bowel syndrome (IBS) is a common disorder that affects the large intestines. It is characterized by pain and cramping within the abdominal region, diarrhea or constipation, gas and bloating food intolerance, and fatigue. The causes of irritable bowel syndrome are multifactorial, and it can be caused by food intolerance, stress, and hormonal imbalance. Studies have shown that many people who have IBS can manage their condition by changing their diet and avoiding foods that may trigger their condition.
- **Inflammatory Bowel Disease:** Although inflammatory bowel disease (IBD) sounds almost the same with IBS, it is crucial to take note that the latter is a type of chronic swelling that affects one or more parts of the digestive tract thus it is not restricted to the large intestines. IBD is accompanied by many kinds of symptoms, including abdominal pain, fatigue, incomplete bowel movements, night sweats, loss of appetite, and rectal bleeding. There are two types of IBD, which include the following:
- **Crohn's Disease:** This type of IBD affects the entire gastrointestinal tract, but it commonly affects the small and large intestines.
- **Ulcerative Colitis:** This type of IBD affects the large intestines only.

Chapter 2: Your Overall Guide to The Low FODMAP Diet

Not too many people have heard of the low FODMAP diet. Unlike other mainstream diets, the FODMAP diet is not as popular as it has only recently been recognized as a diet suitable for people suffering from digestive problems. But what is the low FODMAP diet all about? This chapter will discuss what you need to know about this particular diet regimen.

What Are FODMAPs?

FODMAPs sound foreign to many people, but it is just an acronym for Fermentable Oligo-, Di, Monosaccharides, and Polyols. Don't be confused about its real meaning as it refers to a group of carbohydrates that are known for triggering digestive problems such as stomach pain, gas, and bloating. And as technical as it may sound, FODMAPs are found in a wide variety of foods and varying amounts. Below are different kinds of foods based on the four FODMAPs group.

- **Fermentable** – from the root word ferment, meaning the food can be broken down chemically by microorganisms in the body or gut that commonly involves heat and effervescence or fizz as byproducts.
- **Oligosaccharides** - Oligosaccharides are forms of complex sugar, and they come as fructans and galacto-oligosaccharides. Fructans are sourced from wheat, legumes, and rye. It is also contained in other fruits and vegetables including garlic, green part of onions, savoy cabbage, brussels sprouts, beetroot, artichokes, dandelion leaves. Moreover, prebiotics such as inulin and oligofructose also contain oligosaccharides. On the other hand, Galatians are found in elevated levels from beans, pulses, lentils, tofu, tempeh, and mung beans.
- **Disaccharides** - Disaccharides are two molecules of simple sugars fused together. A good example is lactose.
- **Monosaccharides** - Monosaccharides are simple sugar. They are found in fruits such as figs and mangoes in the form of fructose. Moreover, they are also found in sweeteners such as honey.
- **Polyols** - Polyols refer to organic compounds that contain many hydroxyl groups. Thus, they are neither sugar- nor alcohol-based sweeteners. They are found in fruits – particularly stone fruits such as apples, pears, apricots, peaches, pears, and nectarines, to name a few. They are also found in cauliflower, mushrooms, and many cruciferous vegetables. Low-calorie sweeteners such as xylitol, sorbitol, and mannitol are

examples of polyols. However, certain fruits also contain polyols, including lychee and blackberries.

The Beginnings of The Low FODMAP Diet

The concept of FODMAP has been around only for two decades. In fact, the concept of FODMAP was first introduced in 2005 as part of a research paper by Gibson and Shepherd, which was published in the journal Alimentary Pharmacology & Therapeutics. The paper proposed that reduction of the intake of indigestible short-chained carbohydrates can reduce the stretching or distention of the intestinal wall. The paper aimed to investigate whether this strategy can minimize the stimulation of the gut's nervous system so that people who suffer from IBS can experience relief and alleviation from their condition. When the paper was first proposed, there was no collective term to describe the slowly absorbed and indigestible short-chain carbohydrates. Eventually, the indigestible carbohydrates were identified, and the term FODMAPs as coined to improve the understanding of this concept.

While the concept was introduced in 2005, it was later developed by a team of researchers from Monash University in Melbourne, Australia. It was this research team that undertook the first-ever investigated the role of the FODMAP diet to improve symptoms of functional gastrointestinal disorder, particularly on IBS. Moreover, the university also established an extensive food analysis program in order to identify food and measure the number of FODMAPs that they contain. To date, Monash University is the leading institution that studies FODMAPs on selected Australian and international foods.

Why Do FODMAPs Cause Health Problems?

The thing is that FODMAPs are readily found in nature and people are bound to eat them intentionally or accidentally, are they really bad for the health? They are poorly absorbed in the small intestines; thus, they are eventually fermented by the bacteria, particularly in the distal end of the large intestines. While fermentation of this short-chain is a natural process and results in the production of gas or flatulence, other people may experience excessive bloating. But why do FODMAPs cause a problem for some people? People who are hypersensitive to luminal or stomach distention are affected by FODMAPs. It is essential to take note that the basis of IBS, IBD, and much functional gastrointestinal disorder is the distention of the intestinal lumen that can induce pain, bloating, and motility of the bowel.

Because of this mechanism, therapeutic approaches are designed to reduce distention, particularly on the distal part of the small intestines and the proximal portion of the large intestines. Food that causes distention is poorly absorbed by within the small intestines.

Moreover, they are also osmotically active, which means that draw in more fluid in the body, creating the bloating feeling. Since they are not easily passed as a stool, they are fermented by intestinal bacteria with hydrogen production causing intense bloating.

FODMAPs, specifically fructans, are present in gluten-containing grains; thus, they are also associated with non-celiac gluten sensitivity. The sensitivity may also be manifested as fibromyalgia, dermatitis, and some neurological disorders. While they are associated with IBS and IBD, it is crucial to take note that they do not cause intestinal inflammation. They produce too much gas that can aggravate the condition of people with IBS and IBD thus considering a low FODMAP diet can help avert digestive problems among individuals suffering from functional gastrointestinal disorders in a short period of time.

Understanding the Low FODMAP Diet and Its Benefits

Considering that FODMAPs can aggravate digestive problems, should you eliminate them from your diet? Studies have shown that FODMAPs are also helpful as they produce beneficial alterations within the gut microflora. Avoiding them for a long time can have detrimental effects on the metabolome and gut microbiota. FODMAPs still benefit the body but if you suffer from digestive problems, limiting (and not restricting) your intake is your best option.

Thus, a low FODMAP diet is all about restricting the consumption of foods that are high in FODMAPs and not really completely eliminating them from your body. Limiting the consumption of foods high with FODMAPs have been studied over a population of people who suffer from IBS, and the results have been promising. Below are the benefits of following the low FODMAP diet.

- **Reduced Digestive Problems:** Stomach pain and bloating are the hallmarks of IBS and IBD. Studies have shown that people with IBS experienced significant relief after following a low FODMAP diet. Most of the participants in the study reported 81% of improvement following the diet. Aside from stomach pain, other digestive problems can also be addressed by the FODMAP diet, including flatulence, constipation, and diarrhea.
- **Better Quality Of Life:** Stomach pain and other digestive problems might not be life-threatening, but they can be debilitating. People with IBS often report reduced quality of life, but those who have followed the low FODMAP diet reported stark improvement in their quality of lives. Many also reported that they have more energy following the diet.

Who Is This Diet For?

While a low FODMAP diet can help alleviate digestive problems, this diet is not for everyone. Unless you are diagnosed with IBS or IBD, this diet can bring more harm than benefits. As mentioned earlier, the body still benefits from FODMAPs as they are known prebiotics.

Prebiotics are types of food that can support the growth of good bacteria inside the stomach. Eliminating or limiting its consumption for a long time may cause changes in the gut microflora favoring the proliferation of harmful bacteria. Moreover, while there are many studies on the benefits of a low FODMAP diet among adults with IBS, little is known about its benefits among children with IBS. Thus, there are certain conditions that you have to know if you want to follow this particular diet regimen because even if you have IBS or IBD, you can only do this diet given the following:

- If you have ongoing gut symptoms that are not adequately addressed with your current medication.
- If you have not responded to any types of stress management strategies.
- If you have not responded to first-line advice such as reducing intake of spicy food, alcohol, and caffeine as well as other foods that can commonly trigger stomach problems.

When you try the low FODMAP diet, it is essential to take note that it involves a process. Thus, it is crucial that you carefully observe any changes in your body regardless of whether it is a positive or negative change. Because you need to observe yourself for some time, it is not recommended for first-timers while traveling or while they are going through a stressful or busy period.

Foods to Eat While Following the Low FODMAP Diet

Since the low FODMAP diet limits the intake of food rich in FODMAPs, you must know what kinds of foods that you can eat while following this diet. Below is a list of low FODMAP foods that are categorized by group as analyzed by the Monash University in Australia.

- **Fruits:** Most fruits contain high amounts of FODMAP in the form of fructose. However, some fruits are acceptable in the low FODMAP diet, and these include melon, oranges, and grapes.
- **Vegetables:** Some vegetables contain low amounts of FODMAPs. These include bean sprouts, alfalfa, green beans, bell pepper, bok choy, chives, carrots, zucchini, lettuce, and cucumber.

- **Proteins:** Meats contain protein; thus, they are low in FODMAPs. All meats are included in the low FODMAP diet. However, if you are a vegetarian or a vegan, you can try plant-based protein such as tofu and tempeh because they do not contain too much FODMAPs.
- **Dairy:** Dairy contains lactose which is a type of disaccharide. However, the low FODMAP diet allows dairy as long as they are lactose-free – from milk to yogurt. You can also opt for hard aged cheese as they contain less FODMAPs than other types of cheeses.
- **Bread And Cereals:** Bread, cereals, and pastries that are made from wheat and gluten-rich grains contain high amounts of FODMAPs. Your best alternative is those made from rice, corn, quinoa, potatoes, spelt, and oats.
- **Nuts And Seeds:** Some nuts and seeds contain high amounts of FODMAPs such as cashew and pistachios; thus, it is essential that you choose those that do not come with too much FODMAPs. These include pumpkin seeds and almonds (not more than ten nuts per serving).
- **Beverage:** For your beverage, water is recommended, but you can opt for tea and coffee as long as you do not put sugar in it.

How to Become Successful with The Low FODMAP Diet?

Following the low FODMAP diet is actually more complicated than it sounds. For you to be able to become successful with this diet, there are certain things that you need to do to become successful while following the FODMAP diet.

- **Start Restricting Foods High In Fodmaps:** People who follow the low FODMAP diet think that they need to avoid foods with FODMAP entirely for a long time. Contrary to this false belief, dieters are only recommended to consume small amounts of foods with FODMAP. If you are planning on eliminating FODMAPs in your diet, you should at least do it for three (3) to eight (8) weeks because prolonged restriction can cause detrimental effects to the gut microflora. Thus, the first thing that you need to do is to start restricting eating foods with high FODMAPs content and observe any improvement, if any.
- **Reintroduce Foods High In Fodmaps:** The reason why you need to reintroduce foods rich in FODMAP is to identify the specific types of foods that you can and cannot tolerate. This step is beneficial so that you can establish the types of FODMAPs that you and cannot tolerate. Keeping a diary can be very helpful in this part. In this process, you need to test specific food one by one for three days. You can also work with a trained dietitian to guide you through the process. During this process, you need to follow the low FODMAP diet while you are reintroducing foods high in FODMAPs.

- **Personalize Your Diet:** This is the stage wherein you have to tailor the types of foods that contain FODMAPs according to your personal tolerance. The purpose of this stage is to increase your diet flexibility and variability so that you can achieve long-term compliance and better gut health.

Now that you know that stages that you need to go through to follow a holistic low FODMAP diet, there are several things that you need to know before embarking in this diet. The most important thing to consider is to make sure that you have IBS or IBD. Digestive symptoms may occur in different conditions. Remember that the low FODMAP diet will only work for those with a functional gastrointestinal disorder, particularly IBS.

How to Plan for Your Low FODMAP Diet

The low FODMAP plan may sound simple, but it can be quite challenging to follow, considering that there are so many food items that you have to limit from your diet. This is the reason why it always helps if you plan ahead. This section will give you tips on how to plan ahead if you want to follow the low FODMAP diet.

- **Find Out What To Buy:** Make sure that you have access to low FODMAP foods. You can create a list of what to store on your pantry and scout different grocery stores and farmers market for credible ingredients that are allowed for the low FODMAP diet.
- **Remove All High Fodmap Foods From Your House:** Do an inventory and clear your house – your fridge and pantry – of all foods that contain high FODMAPs. It will not help you with your diet if you have these foods and ingredients still stored around your house.
- **Read Menus Carefully Before Making Your Dishes:** You must familiarize yourself with the low FODMAP menu, especially when you are dining out.

Creating Your Low FODMAP Shopping List

Making a shopping list for your low FODMAP diet purchases is very crucial. This will not only make it easier for you to follow the diet, but it will also make your shopping experience more worthwhile. Below is an example of a shopping list to help you get started with the low FODMAP diet.

- **Whole grains:** Buckwheat, brown rice, corn, oats, millet, and quinoa
- **Protein:** Chicken, beef, fish, pork, lambs, prawns, eggs, and tofu

- **Vegetables:** Bell peppers, bean sprouts, kale, choy sum, carrots, spinach, tomatoes, and zucchini
- **Fruits:** Blueberries, bananas, lime, kiwi, oranges, any citrus fruits, pineapple, papaya, and strawberries
- **Seeds:** Pumpkin seeds, sesame seeds, sunflower seeds, linseed
- **Nuts:** Macadamia nuts, peanuts, pine nuts, pecans, walnuts, and almonds (10 almonds only per day).
- **Dairy:** Lactose-free milk, cheddar cheese, and parmesan cheese
- **Oils:** Olive oil and coconut oil
- **Condiments:** Chili pepper, basil, mustard, ginger, salt and pepper, mustard, wasabi powder, saffron, turmeric, and rice vinegar
- **Beverages:** Water, coffee, black tea, green tea, white tea, peppermint tea

When you buy ingredients, it is not only essential to check their face value as food companies may add FODMAPS to their food as a fat substitute and improve the prebiotic qualities of their products. It will be helpful if you opt for foods that are not processed to avoid these unnecessary additions.

Low FODMAP Diet FAQs

Q1: Is The Low FODMAP Diet Less Flavorful Than Others Because You Cannot Use Onions And Garlic?

You may be omitting onions and garlic from the low FODMAP diet, but this does not mean that the food you make is less flavorful. There are many spices and herbs that you can still use to improve the flavor of your meals.

Q2: Can Vegetarians Follow The Low FODMAP Diet?

A well-balanced vegetarian diet can also be low in FODMAPs, but it can be more challenging because the legumes that are a staple to any vegetarian diet as protein alternatives among many vegetarians are high in FODMAPs. Having said this, you can still include small portions of legumes (about 64 grams) as long as they are canned or soaked in water and rinsed.

Q3: What if My Symptoms Don't Improve After Following The Low FODMAP Diet?

It is vital to take note that the low FODMAP diet does not work for everyone who suffers from IBS. In fact, studies show that approximately 30% of people with IBS do not respond well to this diet. You can talk to your doctor about other alternative options that you can take.

Chapter 3 Low FODMAP Breakfast Recipes

Mini Banana Pancakes

Prep time: 10 minutes, Cook time: 6 minutes; Serves: 4

Ingredients:

- 2 small bananas
- 2 large eggs
- 2 tablespoon gluten-free all-purpose flour
- ½ teaspoon ground cinnamon
- ¼ teaspoon ground nutmeg

What you' ll need from the store cupboard:

- 1 tablespoon brown sugar
- ¼ teaspoon baking powder
- 1/8 teaspoon salt

Instructions:

1. In a large bowl, peel and mash the bananas until smooth. Whisk in the eggs until well combined before adding the gluten-free flour, cinnamon, and nutmeg.
2. Add in brown sugar, baking powder, and salt.
3. Heat a non-stick frying pan over medium flame and scoop a batter into the pan.
4. Allow the batter to cook until small bubbles form on top.
5. Flip over the pancake and cook until the other side turns golden brown.

Nutrition Facts Per Serving:

Calories 96, Total Fat 2.5g, Saturated Fat 0.9g, Total Carbs 17.3g, Net Carbs 15g, Protein 2.3g, Sugar: 8.1g, Fiber: 1.2g, Sodium: 83mg, Potassium: 229mg

Dark Chocolate Granola

Prep time: 10 minutes, **Cook time:** 20 minutes; **Serves:** 16

Ingredients:

- 2 cups quinoa flakes
- 1 cup sunflower and pumpkin seeds
- ½ cup coconut chips, dehydrated
- 6 tablespoons cocoa powder
- 6 tablespoons olive oil

What you'll need from the store cupboard:

- 4 tablespoons pure maple syrup
- 1 teaspoon vanilla extract
- 1/8 teaspoon salt

Instructions:

1. Preheat the oven to 250 °F for 5 minutes.
2. In a bowl, mix together the ingredients until well combined.
3. Spread the granola mixture over baking tray lined with parchment paper.
4. Bake in the oven for at least 20 minutes.
5. Halfway through the cooking time, stir the granola to cook evenly.
6. Once cooked, take out from the oven and allow to cool for two hours before serving or storing in air-tight containers.

Nutrition Facts Per Serving:

Calories 207, Total Fat 12.2g, Saturated Fat 2.3g, Total Carbs 21.3g, Net Carbs 18.3g, Protein 5.3g, Sugar: 4.5g, Fiber: 3g, Sodium: 30mg, Potassium: 248mg

Breakfast Muesli

Prep time: 10 minutes, **Cook time:** 15 minutes; **Serves:** 6

Ingredients:

- 5 cups gluten-free cornflakes
- 1 ½ cups quinoa puffs
- 7 tablespoons dried shredded coconut
- 4 tablespoons pumpkin seeds
- 15 banana chips, crushed

What you' ll need from the store cupboard:

- 6 tablespoons olive oil
- 1/3 cup brown sugar

Instructions:

1. Preheat the oven to 300⁰F.
2. Place the cornflakes in a plastic bag and crush using a rolling pin.
3. In a bowl, put the cornflakes, quinoa puffs, coconut, pumpkin seeds, and banana chips. Stir in the olive oil and brown sugar. Mix until well combined.
4. Spread the mixture over a baking sheet lined with parchment paper.
5. Bake in the oven for 15 minutes while tossing every 10 minutes for even cooking.
6. Once cooked, allow to cool before placing muesli in an airtight container.

Nutrition Facts Per Serving:

Calories 464, Total Fat 19.5g, Saturated Fat 3.1g, Total Carbs 62.9g, Net Carbs 56.3g, Protein 11.2g, Sugar: 12.6g, Fiber: 6.6g, Sodium: 241mg, Potassium: 249mg

Quinoa Porridge with Berries

Prep time: 5 minutes, Cook time: 20 minutes; Serves: 2

Ingredients:

- ½ cup quinoa
- ¾ cup coconut milk
- ¼ teaspoon ground cinnamon
- 4 teaspoons pure maple syrup
- 1 cup fresh berries of your choice

What you'll need from the store cupboard:

- 1 teaspoon oil
- 1 cup water

Instructions:

1. Place quinoa in a sieve and rinse under running water for at least 2 minutes.
2. Place in a saucepan and add oil. Toast over medium heat or until the quinoa has turned brown.
3. Pour over a cup of water and bring to a boil. Allow to simmer for 15 minutes. The quinoa is cooked once it becomes fluffy. Drain off excess water and return the quinoa to the pan.
4. Pour in coconut milk, cinnamon, and maple syrup.
5. Allow the porridge to simmer for 5 minutes.
6. Pour in the berries before serving.

Nutrition Facts Per Serving:

Calories 441, Total Fat 26.5g, Saturated Fat 19.6g, Total Carbs 46.8g, Net Carbs 40.2g, Protein 8.6g, Sugar: 14.5g, Fiber: 6.6g, Sodium: 20mg, Potassium: 615mg

Salmon and Spinach Omelet

Ingredients:

- 6 large eggs
- 1 ½ tablespoons coconut milk
- 1/8 teaspoon paprika
- 1 can canned salmons, flaked
- 2 cups spinach
- ½ cup cherry tomatoes, halved

What you' ll need from the store cupboard:

- salt and pepper to taste
- 2 teaspoons sunflower oil

Instructions:

1. In a bowl, whisk together the eggs and coconut milk until well combined. Season with salt and pepper to taste.
2. Heat a pan over medium flame and add sunflower oil.
3. Pour the egg mixture and sprinkle with paprika on top and add in the salmon flakes and spinach.
4. Allow to set then flip the omelet and cook until the spinach becomes wilted.
5. Serve and top with cherry tomatoes.

Nutrition Facts Per Serving:

Calories 556, Total Fat 35.8g, Saturated Fat 10.8g, Total Carbs 6.1g, Net Carbs 4.8g, Protein 52.7g, Sugar: 2.2g, Fiber: 1.3g, Sodium: 954mg, Potassium: 1023mg

"Baked Beans" With Egg on Toast

Prep time: 3 minutes, **Cook time:** 5 minutes; **Serves:** 1

Ingredients:

- ¼ cup canned chickpeas, drained and rinsed
- ¼ cup tomato, blended
- 1/8 teaspoon paprika powder
- 1/8 teaspoon Worcestershire sauce
- 1 egg
- 1 slice gluten-free bread, toasted
- 1 handful rocket arugula

What you'll need from the store cupboard:

- Salt and pepper to taste

Instructions:

1. In a bowl, combine the chickpeas and tomatoes. Add in paprika and Worcestershire sauce. Season with salt and pepper to taste.
2. Turn on the stove and cook for 5 minutes. Set aside.
3. Heat a non-stick frying pan and crack open the egg into the pan. Cook until the eggs have set.
4. Assemble the toast by putting on top of the bread the beans. Top the beans with egg and arugula last.

Nutrition Facts Per Serving:

Calories 276, Total Fat 11.6g, Saturated Fat 4.9g, Total Carbs 28.2g, Net Carbs 23.3g, Protein 15.6g, Sugar: 7.1g, Fiber: 4.9g, Sodium: 221mg, Potassium: 628mg

Breakfast Wraps

Ingredients:

- 2 large eggs, beaten
- 1 ½ teaspoons chopped fresh chives
- ½ cup baby spinach
- ½ medium tomato, sliced
- A half of an avocado, pitted and flesh scooped out

What you' ll need from the store cupboard:

- A tiny amount of oil
- Salt and pepper to taste

Instructions:

1. Heat oil in a frying pan over medium heat.
2. In a bowl, whisk the eggs and season with salt and pepper to taste.
3. Pour the egg mixture into the pan and cook as you would a pancake. Carefully flip the egg to avoid breaking.
4. Set aside to cool.
5. Place the egg on a plate and put chives, spinach, tomato, and avocado on one side of the egg.
6. Fold carefully to avoid breaking the egg.

Nutrition Facts Per Serving:

Calories 294, Total Fat 24g, Saturated Fat 5.4g, Total Carbs 15g, Net Carbs 7.1g, Protein 8.9g, Sugar: 3.4g, Fiber: 7.9g, Sodium: 39mg, Potassium: 783mg

Chapter 4 Low FODMAP Smoothie Recipes

Blueberry Lime Coconut Smoothie

Prep time: 2 minutes, Cook time: 0 minutes; Serves: 1

Ingredients:

- ½ cup fresh or frozen blueberries
- 2 tablespoons flaked coconut
- 2 tablespoons fresh lime juice
- 4 ounces lactose-free yogurt
- 1 teaspoon chia seeds
- 1 cup ice

What you' ll need from the store cupboard:

- None

Instructions:

1. Place all ingredients in a blender.
2. Pulse until smooth.
3. Serve immediately.

Nutrition Facts Per Serving:

Calories 120, Total Fat 1g, Saturated Fat 0.2g, Total Carbs 17g, Net Carbs 14.5g, Protein 12.2g, Sugar: 11.5g, Fiber: 2.5g, Sodium: 74mg, Potassium: 312mg

Strawberry Smoothie

Ingredients:

- ½ cup coconut milk
- 1 can fresh strawberries
- ¼ cup vanilla soy ice cream
- 1 ½ teaspoon rice protein powder
- 1 teaspoon chia seeds
- ½ tablespoon maple syrup
- 1 teaspoon lemon juice
- 6 ice cubes

What you'll need from the store cupboard:

- None

Instructions:

1. Place all ingredients in a blender.
2. Pulse until smooth.
3. Serve while still cold.

Nutrition Facts Per Serving:

Calories 168, Total Fat 4.1g, Saturated Fat 0.5g, Total Carbs 21.4g, Net Carbs 15.4g, Protein 13.9g, Sugar: 11.2g, Fiber: 6g, Sodium: 75mg, Potassium: 353mg

Oatmeal Cookie Breakfast Smoothie

Prep time: 2 minutes, **Cook time:** 0 minutes; **Serves:** 1

Ingredients:

- 1 yellow banana, peeled and sliced
- ¾ cup almond milk
- ¼ cup ice
- 1/8 tablespoon vanilla
- ½ teaspoon cinnamon powder
- 2 tablespoons rolled oats
- A dash of ground nutmeg

What you'll need from the store cupboard:

- None

Instructions:

1. Place all ingredients in a blender.
2. Pulse until smooth.
3. Serve immediately.

Nutrition Facts Per Serving:

Calories 303, Total Fat 7.8g, Saturated Fat 2.5g, Total Carbs 60g, Net Carbs 52.1g, Protein 5.5g, Sugar: 32.6g, Fiber: 7.9g, Sodium: 146mg, Potassium: 698mg

Green Kiwi Smoothie

Ingredients:

- 1 cup seedless green grapes
- 1 kiwi, peeled and chopped
- 2 tablespoons water
- 8 inches cucumber, cut into chunks
- 2 cups baby spinach
- 1 ½ cups ice cubes
- 1 green apple, peeled and cored

What you' ll need from the store cupboard:

- None

Instructions:

1. Place all ingredients in a blender.
2. Pulse until the mixture becomes smooth.
3. Serve immediately.

Nutrition Facts Per Serving:

Calories 132, Total Fat 1 g, Saturated Fat 0.5g, Total Carbs 33g, Net Carbs 30g, Protein 3g, Sugar: 25g, Fiber: 3g, Sodium: 4mg, Potassium: 226mg

Pumpkin Smoothie

Prep time: 2 minutes, **Cook time:** 0 minutes; **Serves:** 1

Ingredients:

- ½ frozen medium ripe bananas, peeled and sliced
- ¼ cup pumpkin puree
- ½ cup coconut milk
- ¼ teaspoon pumpkin pie spice
- 1 tablespoon maple syrup
- ½ cup crushed ice
- A pinch of cinnamon

What you' ll need from the store cupboard:

- None

Instructions:

1. Place all ingredients in a blender except for the cinnamon.
2. Blend until smooth.
3. Put into glasses and sprinkle with cinnamon before serving.

Nutrition Facts Per Serving:

Calories 695, Total Fat 37.7g, Saturated Fat 30g, Total Carbs 52.3g, Net Carbs 43.1g, Protein 14.3g, Sugar: 29.6g, Fiber: 9.2g, Sodium: 56mg, Potassium: 829mg

Chocolate Sesame Smoothie

Prep time: 2 minutes, Cook time: 0 minutes; Serves: 1

Ingredients:

- 1 tablespoon sesame seeds
- 2 teaspoons unsweetened raw cocoa powder
- Half of a medium banana, peeled and sliced
- Flesh from 1/8 slice of avocado
- 1 tablespoon maple syrup
- 1 cup coconut milk
- ½ cup ice

What you'll need from the store cupboard:

- None

Instructions:

1. Place all ingredients in a blender.
2. Pulse until smooth.
3. Pour in a glass and serve immediately.

Nutrition Facts Per Serving:

Calories 406, Total Fat 17.5g, Saturated Fat 6.3g, Total Carbs 57.3g, Net Carbs 50.5g, Protein 11.8g, Sugar: 39.2g, Fiber: 6.8g, Sodium: 115mg, Potassium: 1033mg

Chapter 5 Low FODMAP Snack Recipes

Sponge Cake

Prep time: 15 minutes, **Cook time:** 20 minutes; **Serves:** 8

Ingredients:

- 4 eggs
- 1 tablespoon boiling water
- ¾ cup granulated sugar
- 1 cup cornstarch
- 1tablespoon gluten-free all-purpose flour
- 2 teaspoon baking powder
- 4 tablespoon strawberry jam
- 1 cup fresh strawberries

What you' ll need from the store cupboard:

- Butter for greasing cake pan

Instructions:

1. Preheat the oven to 355^{0}F.
2. Grease a cake pan with butter and set aside.
3. Separate the egg whites from the yolk. Beat the yolks and set aside.
4. Whisk the egg whites using an eggbeater and gradually add boiling water. Beat until the egg whites form stiff peaks. Add sugar gradually until everything is dissolved. Fold in gently the beaten egg yolks.
5. Sift the cornstarch, gluten-free flour, and baking powder. Sift into another bowl.
6. Add the dry ingredients into the egg mixture until well-combined.
7. Pour cake batter into prepared cake pan and bake for 20 minutes or until a toothpick inserted in the middle comes out clean.
8. Allow the cake to cool before removing from the cake pan.
9. Spread jam on top of the cake and arrange strawberry slices.

Nutrition Facts Per Serving:

Calories 179, Total Fat 4.9g, Saturated Fat 1.2g, Total Carbs 28.5g, Net Carbs 27.8g, Protein 4.7g, Sugar: 12.1g, Fiber: 0.7g, Sodium: 53mg, Potassium: 114mg

Roasted Rhubarb with Custard and Ginger Crumbs

Prep time: 15 minutes, Cook time: 15 minutes; Serves: 4

Ingredients:

- ½ cup fresh rhubarb cut into 2-inches pieces
- 6 soft ginger cookies
- A dash of ground cinnamon
- 1/8 teaspoon ground ginger
- 2 tablespoon custard powder
- ½ teaspoon vanilla extract
- 2 cups almond milk

What you'll need from the store cupboard:

- 2 tablespoons white sugar
- 1 tablespoon brown sugar

Instructions:

1. Preheat the oven to 355^0F.
2. Line a roasting tray with baking paper and arrange the rhubarb in the prepared tray. Sprinkle with a tablespoon of white sugar. Roast for 15 minutes until the rhubarb is tender.
3. Meanwhile, make the ginger crumbs and the custard.
4. In a bowl, crumble the ginger cookies and place the brown sugar, cinnamon, and ginger. Place on a tray and bake for another 12 minutes for 12 minutes.
5. Make the custard by combining the custard powder, remaining white sugar, vanilla extract, and milk. Cook in the microwave and heat for 3 minutes.
6. Assemble the roasted rhubarb by topping it with custard and ginger crumbs.

Nutrition Facts Per Serving:

Calories 224, Total Fat 7.1g, Saturated Fat 3.1g, Total Carbs 36.5g, Net Carbs 35.6g, Protein 4.9g, Sugar: 31.4g, Fiber: 0.9g, Sodium: 147mg, Potassium: 223mg

Sunshine Popsicle

Prep time: 8 hours, Cook time: 0 minutes; Serves: 4

Ingredients:

- 4 large carrots, peeled and grated
- 3 large oranges
- 1 teaspoon orange zest
- 1 imperial mandarin, peeled and chopped finely

What you' ll need from the store cupboard:

- None

Instructions:

1. Place the grated carrots in a clean cloth and squeeze until the juices of the carrots are squeezed out.
2. Place the squeezed-out juice of the carrots in a bowl. Add in the orange zest and the orange juice. Stir in the chopped imperial mandarin.
3. Pour into popsicle molds and freeze overnight.

Nutrition Facts Per Serving:

Calories 90, Total Fat 0.5g, Saturated Fat 0g, Total Carbs 22.1g, Net Carbs 17.1g, Protein 1.6g, Sugar: 15.5g, Fiber: 5g, Sodium: 50mg, Potassium: 448mg

Frozen Strawberry and Banana Bars with Chocolate Fudge Sauce

Prep time: 10 minutes, Cook time: 5 minutes; Serves: 4

Ingredients:

- 2 small frozen bananas
- 1 cup frozen strawberries
- 5 tablespoons coconut yoghurt
- 2 tablespoon maple syrup
- 1 teaspoon vanilla extract
- 3 tablespoons coconut milk
- ¼ cup dark chocolate
- 1 ½ tablespoon cocoa powder
- 2 tablespoons maple syrup

What you'll need from the store cupboard:

- None

Instructions:

1. Place the frozen bananas, strawberries, yoghurt, maple syrup, and vanilla extract in a blender and pulse until smooth.
2. Place in a lidded container and allow to freeze overnight.
3. Meanwhile, prepare the chocolate fudge sauce by heating in a saucepan the coconut milk, dark chocolate, cocoa powder, and maple syrup. Cook on low heat for 5 minutes or until the sauce thickens. Set aside until the frozen fruit mixture is ready.
4. Slice the frozen fruit into bars and pour over the chocolate sauce.

Nutrition Facts Per Serving:

Calories 217, Total Fat 4.1g, Saturated Fat 2.4g, Total Carbs 44.3g, Net Carbs 37.7g, Protein 3.8g, Sugar:29.1g, Fiber: 6.6g, Sodium: 281mg, Potassium: 1082mg

Frozen Berry Yoghurt Bark

Ingredients:

- 2 cups strawberries
- 2 cups blueberries
- 2 cups raspberries
- 2 cups coconut yoghurt
- 2 tablespoons strawberry jam
- 1 teaspoon vanilla extract

What you'll need from the store cupboard:

- None

Instructions:

1. Line a baking tray with parchment paper.
2. Chop the berries and arrange them on a baking tray.
3. Spread the yoghurt into the baking tray. Make sure that the yoghurt is thick enough to cover the strawberries.
4. Swirl in the strawberry jam and sprinkle with vanilla extract.
5. Place in the fridge to freeze.

Once frozen, cut haphazardly using a knife to resemble barks.

Nutrition Facts Per Serving:

Calories 262, Total Fat 15.4g, Saturated Fat 5.5g, Total Carbs 32.9g, Net Carbs 21.1g, Protein 3.6g, Sugar: 17.5g, Fiber: 11.8g, Sodium: 11mg, Potassium 430 mg

Salted Pumpkin Seeds with Caramel Sauce

Prep time: 0 minutes, Cook time: 25 minutes; Serves: 16

Ingredients:

- 2 cups pumpkin seeds, hulled
- ¼ teaspoon ground cinnamon
- ½ teaspoon ground ginger
- 1/8 teaspoon ground nutmeg
- 2 ½ tablespoons white sugar

What you'll need from the store cupboard:

- 1 tablespoon olive oil
- 2 ½ tablespoons brown sugar
- 2 teaspoons water
- ½ teaspoon rock salt

Instructions:

1. Preheat the oven to 300^0F.
2. In a bowl, mix together the pumpkin seeds, cinnamon, ginger, and nutmeg. Add in white sugar and water.
3. Line the roasting tray with baking paper and spread the pumpkin seeds on the tray. Bake for 25 minutes until the pumpkin seeds are golden and crunchy.
4. While the pumpkin seeds are baking, make the caramel sauce. Combine the olive oil, brown sugar, and water.
5. Cook over medium flame until the sugar dissolves.
6. Once the pumpkin seeds are cooked, drizzle the caramel sauce and mix. Sprinkle with salt last.

Nutrition Facts Per Serving:

Calories 94, Total Fat 8.2g, Saturated Fat 1.2g, Total Carbs 3.1g, Net Carbs 2.1g, Protein 4.4g, Sugar: 0.9g, Fiber: 1g, Sodium: 38mg, Potassium: 119mg

Chapter 6 Low FODMAP Seafood Recipes

Gluten-Free Fried Fish

Prep time: 10 minutes, Cook time: 8 minutes; Serves: 2

Ingredients:

- 1 cup white rice flour
- 1 egg, lightly beaten
- 1 cup mashed potato flakes
- 1 lb. white fish of your choice, filleted
- 2 tablespoons olive oil
- 2 tablespoons butter

What you'll need from the store cupboard:

- salt and pepper to taste

Instructions:

1. Put in individual bowls the rice flour, egg, and mashed potato flakes.
2. Dip the fish fillets in rice flour, egg, and mashed potato flakes. Season with salt and pepper to taste.
3. In a large skillet heated over medium flame, add oil and butter and fry the fish for 4 minutes on each side.

Nutrition Facts Per Serving:

Calories 791, Total Fat 31.4g, Saturated Fat 10.7g, Total Carbs 79.4g, Net Carbs 75.5g, Protein 45.2g, Sugar: 2.6g, Fiber: 3.9g, Sodium:942 mg, Potassium: 1082mg

Spicy Lemon Shrimps

Prep time: 5 minutes, **Cook time:** 6 minutes; **Serves:** 1

Ingredients:

- 2 tablespoons butter
- 1 ¼ pounds uncooked large shrimps, peeled and deveined
- Juice from ½ lemon
- ¼ teaspoon red pepper flakes
- 4 cups spinach

What you'll need from the store cupboard:

- Salt and pepper to taste

Instructions:

1. Heat the butter in a skillet and place the shrimps, lemon juice, and red pepper flakes. Season with salt and pepper to taste.
2. Stir in the spinach and continue cooking until the spinach has wilted. Cook for 6 minutes otherwise the shrimps will become overcooked.
3. Serve immediately.

Nutrition Facts Per Serving:

Calories 644, Total Fat 29.2g, Saturated Fat 16.2g, Total Carbs 12.3g, Net Carbs 9.4g, Protein 81.1g, Sugar: 1.7g, Fiber: 2.9g, Sodium: 344mg, Potassium: 1389mg

Seafood in Coconut Sauce

Prep time: 5 minutes, **Cook time:** 6 minutes; **Serves:** 4

Ingredients:

- 1 tablespoon coconut oil
- 1 teaspoon minced ginger
- 1 cup mussel meat
- ½ cup crab meat, shredded
- ½ cup prawns, peeled and deveined
- 1 cup coconut cream
- 1 lemongrass stalk

What you' ll need from the store cupboard:

- Salt and paper to taste

Instructions:

1. In a large skillet, heat the oil and sauté the ginger for a minute.
2. Stir in the mussels, crab meat, and prawns.
3. Add in the coconut cream and lemon grass.
4. Allow to cook for 6 minutes or until the prawns are done.

Nutrition Facts Per Serving:

Calories 341, Total Fat 25.3g, Saturated Fat 21.4g, Total Carbs 18.7g, Net Carbs 11.5g, Protein 15.7g, Sugar: 0.2g, Fiber: 7.2g, Sodium: 14mg, Potassium: 398mg

England Shrimp Boil

Prep time: 5 minutes, Cook time: 8 minutes; Serves: 12

Ingredients:

- 2 tablespoons olive oil
- 1 tablespoon fennel seed
- 1 tablespoon mustard seed
- ½ teaspoon red pepper flakes
- 3 12-oz bottles of beer
- 1 lemon, quartered
- 3 lbs. fresh shrimps, heads off and shells on
- ½ cup unsalted butter

What you'll need from the store cupboard:

- salt and pepper to taste

Instructions:

1. In a deep pot, heat the oil and add in the fennel seeds and mustard seeds until toasted. Add in the red pepper flakes and season with salt and pepper to taste.
2. Pour in the beer then squeeze the lemon wedges into the pot.
3. Add in the shrimps and bring to a boil for 4 minutes.
4. Drain the shrimps and discard the liquid.
5. Pile the shrimps in a platter and top with butter before serving.

Nutrition Facts Per Serving:

Calories 186, Total Fat 9.2g, Saturated Fat 3.7g, Total Carbs 0.9g, Net Carbs 0.6g, Protein 23.7g, Sugar: 0.2g, Fiber: 0.3g, Sodium: 992mg, Potassium: 120mg

Cacciuto

Prep time: 4 minutes, Cook time: 8 minutes; Serves: 4

Ingredients:

- 1 tablespoon olive oil
- 1 small fennel bulb, peeled and sliced thinly
- 2 medium sized carrots, peeled and chopped
- 1 cup white wine
- 4 small filleted white fish
- 1 cup prawn meat
- Lemon cut into wedges

What you' ll need from the store cupboard:

- Salt and pepper to taste

Instructions:

1. Heat the oil in a pot over medium flame and sauté the fennel bulb and carrots for 5 minutes until tender.
2. Add in the white wine and allow to simmer for 3 minutes.
3. Add in the fish fillet and prawn meat. Season with salt and pepper to taste.
4. Serve with lemon wedges.

Nutrition Facts Per Serving:

Calories 282, Total Fat 7.9g, Saturated Fat 1.3g, Total Carbs 17.1g, Net Carbs 10.5g, Protein 36.3g, Sugar: 4.7g, Fiber: 6.6g, Sodium: 112mg, Potassium: 1426mg

Seafood Adobo

Ingredients:

- 1 tablespoon olive oil
- 1 medium red pepper, diced
- 1 tablespoon adobo seasoning
- 2 cups blend of calamari, scallops, and shrimps
- 1/3 cup green olives, chopped
- Juice from ½ lemon

What you'll need from the store cupboard:

- Salt and pepper to taste

Instructions:

1. Heat the oil in a pan over medium flame.
2. Sauté the red pepper and add in the adobo seasoning for 30 seconds.
3. Stir in the sea-foods and green olives.
4. Add in lemon juice and season with salt and pepper to taste.
5. Allow to cook for 6 minutes until the sea-foods are done.

Nutrition Facts Per Serving:

Calories 122, Total Fat 5.9g, Saturated Fat 1.8g, Total Carbs 14.6g, Net Carbs 13.7g, Protein 2.7g, Sugar: 12.9g, Fiber: 0.9g, Sodium: 195mg, Potassium: 207mg

Grilled Halibut

Prep time: 60 minutes, Cook time: 8 minutes; Serves: 1

Ingredients:

- 1 12-ounces halibut fillet
- 2 tablespoons lemon juice
- A dash of red pepper flakes
- Chopped parsley for garnish

What you' ll need from the store cupboard:

- Salt and pepper to taste

Instructions:

1. Place the halibut in a bowl and add in all ingredients except for the parsley.
2. Allow to marinate for about 1 hour inside the fridge.
3. Heat the grill to medium high.
4. Once hot, place the halibut on the grill rack and cook for 4 minutes on each side or until the fish is flaky.
5. Garnish with chopped parsley before serving.

Nutrition Facts Per Serving:

Calories 679, Total Fat 47.7g, Saturated Fat 8.3g, Total Carbs 10.2g, Net Carbs 7.5g, Protein 51.6g, Sugar: 3.6g, Fiber: 2.7g, Sodium: 309mg, Potassium: 1429mg

Chapter 7 Low FODMAP Poultry Recipes

Maple Mustard Chicken with Rosemary

Prep time: 5 minutes, **Cook time:** 35 minutes; **Serves:** 6

Ingredients:

- 1 tablespoon olive oil
- 6 bone-in chicken thighs
- 2 tablespoons Dijon mustard
- 2 tablespoons whole grain mustard seed
- 3 tablespoons maple syrup
- 1 tablespoon lemon juice
- 1 tablespoon fresh rosemary

What you' ll need from the store cupboard:

- Salt and pepper to taste

Instructions:

1. Preheat the oven to 375^{0}F and grease a baking dish.
2. Season the chicken thighs with salt and pepper to taste.
3. Heat the oil in a large skillet over medium flame and put the chicken thighs skin side down and cook for 4 minutes on each side or until the skin turns golden brown.
4. While the chicken is cooking on the stovetop, prepare the mustard glaze by mixing the rest of the ingredients in a bowl.
5. Once the chicken has turned golden, transfer into the prepared baking dish.
6. Brush each thigh with the prepared mustard sauce.
7. Place inside the oven and bake for 30 minutes or until the chicken is cooked through.

Nutrition Facts Per Serving:

Calories 487, Total Fat 35.2g, Saturated Fat 9.1g, Total Carbs 8.3g, Net Carbs 7.8g, Protein 32.6g, Sugar: 6.3g, Fiber: 0.5g, Sodium: 215mg, Potassium: 443mg

Baked Potato and Chicken Casserole

Prep time: 10 minutes, Cook time: 35 minutes; Serves: 4

Ingredients:

- 4 medium russet potatoes, scrubbed and diced
- 1 lb. boneless chicken breasts, skin removed and diced
- 4 slices of bacon, cooked crisp and crumbled
- ½ cup coconut cream
- 1 ½ cups cheddar cheese, grated
- 4 green onions, green parts chopped

What you'll need from the store cupboard:

- salt and pepper to taste

Instructions:

1. Heat the oven to 350^{0}F and grease a casserole pan.
2. Spread the potatoes in the bottom of the pan. Place the chicken on top and season with salt and pepper to taste.
3. Sprinkle with bacon crumbles.
4. Pour in the coconut cream and top with cheddar cheese, and green onions.
5. Place inside the oven and bake for 35 minutes

Nutrition Facts Per Serving:

Calories 662, Total Fat 35.4g, Saturated Fat 14.7g, Total Carbs 49.3g, Net Carbs g, Protein 38.9g, Sugar: 7.3g, Fiber: 4.7g, Sodium: 685mg, Potassium: 1153mg

Quick Curry Casserole

Prep time: 10 minutes, **Cook time:** 20 minutes; **Serves:** 4

Ingredients:

- 2 chicken breasts
- 2 cups broccoli florets
- ½ cup Mayonnaise
- 2 teaspoons curry powder
- 1 teaspoon lemon juice
- 1 bell pepper, seeded and chopped
- 1 cup grated cheese

What you'll need from the store cupboard:

- Oil for frying
- Salt and pepper to taste

Instructions:

1. Heat the oven to 375^0F and grease the casserole dish.
2. Heat the oil in a large pan and fry the chicken breasts on each side until golden brown. Set aside.
3. Using the same pan, cook the broccoli florets for 2 minutes. Set aside.
4. In a bowl, combine the mayonnaise, curry powder, and lemon juice. Season with the salt and pepper to taste.
5. Place the chicken in the casserole dish and top with broccoli.
6. Pour over the curry sauce and top with bell pepper and cheese.
7. Bake in the oven for 15 minutes.

Nutrition Facts Per Serving:

Calories 482, Total Fat 33.2g, Saturated Fat 11g, Total Carbs 3.4g, Net Carbs 1.8g, Protein 41.1g, Sugar: 1.1g, Fiber: 1.6g, Sodium: 529mg, Potassium: 465mg

One Pan Chicken Cacciatore

Prep time: 10 minutes, Cook time: 25 minutes; Serves: 4

Ingredients:

- 2 tablespoons olive oil
- 2 pounds boneless chicken thighs
- 2 small carrots, sliced thinly
- 1 red bell pepper, seeded and diced
- ¼ teaspoon red pepper flakes
- ½ cup dry red wine
- 2 tablespoons pitted Kalamata olives
- 2 cups crushed tomatoes
- 4 sprigs fresh thyme, chopped
- 4 sprigs fresh oregano, chopped

What you' ll need from the store cupboard:

- Salt and pepper to taste

Instructions:

1. In a skillet, heat the oil over medium flame. Season the chicken thighs with salt and pepper to taste and cook the chicken until golden brown. Remove from the plate and set aside.
2. On the same skillet, sauté the vegetables and scrape the brown bits at the bottom of the pan. Continue cooking for 5 minutes and season the vegetables with salt and pepper to taste.
3. Pour in the red wine and simmer until reduced by half. Add the olives, tomatoes, thyme, and oregano. Place the chicken on top of the vegetables.
4. Allow to simmer for 15 minutes.

Nutrition Facts Per Serving:

Calories 591, Total Fat 45.1g, Saturated Fat 11.3g, Total Carbs 5.2g, Net Carbs 3.9g, Protein 28.5g, Sugar: 2.8g, Fiber: 1.3g, Sodium: 223mg, Potassium: 702mg

Moroccan Chicken

Prep time: 8 hours, **Cook time:** 16 minutes; **Serves:** 4

Ingredients:

- 2 tablespoons olive oil
- 2 teaspoons ground paprika
- 1 teaspoon ground cumin
- ½ teaspoon ground coriander
- ½ teaspoon ground turmeric
- ¼ teaspoon ground ginger
- 1/8 teaspoon cayenne pepper
- 1 package 20-oz boneless and skinless chicken breasts

What you'll need from the store cupboard:

- Salt and pepper to taste

Instructions:

1. In a bowl, combine all ingredients except for the chicken.
2. Place the chicken breasts in a Ziploc bag and pour in the sauce. Allow to marinate in the fridge for at least 8 hours.
3. Heat the grill to medium and remove the chicken from the marinade.
4. Grill the chicken for 8 minutes on each side until fully cooked.

Nutrition Facts Per Serving:

Calories 237, Total Fat 10.2g, Saturated Fat 1.8g, Total Carbs 1.2g, Net Carbs 1g, Protein 32.2g, Sugar:0.1g, Fiber: 0.2g, Sodium: 66mg, Potassium: 520mg

Chicken Pub Rub

Prep time: 10 minutes, **Cook time:** 30 minutes; **Serves:** 4

Ingredients:

- 4 chicken breasts, bone in
- 1 teaspoon dried basil
- 1 teaspoon dried rosemary
- ½ teaspoon mustard powder
- ½ teaspoon paprika
- ½ teaspoon dried thyme
- ¼ teaspoon celery seed
- 1/8 teaspoon ground cumin
- 1/8 teaspoon cayenne pepper

What you' ll need from the store cupboard:

- Salt and pepper to taste

Instructions:

1. Preheat the oven to 350^0F and grease a baking dish.
2. Place all ingredients in a bowl and mix until the chicken is coated with the condiments.
3. Place the chicken in the baking dish. Cover the dish with foil to prevent the chicken from drying out.
4. Cook for 30 minutes until the internal temperature of the chicken reaches 205^0F.

Nutrition Facts Per Serving:

Calories 502, Total Fat 26.9g, Saturated Fat 7.7g, Total Carbs 0.5g, Net Carbs 0.2g, Protein 60.6g, Sugar: 0.05g, Fiber: 0.3g, Sodium: 190mg, Potassium: 656mg

Thai Green Curried Chicken

Prep time: 10 minutes, Cook time:15 minutes; Serves: 8

Ingredients:

- 2 stalks lemon grass
- 4 green chilies
- 6 spring onions, green part only
- 1 tablespoon grated ginger
- ½ cup fresh coriander
- ½ cup fresh basil
- 1 teaspoon ground cumin
- 1 teaspoon fish sauce
- Zest from one lemon
- 2 tablespoons coconut oil
- 1 ½ chicken breasts, cut into bite-sized pieces
- 1 can coconut milk
- 2 sweet peppers, cut into strips
- ¾ cup baby corn, sliced

What you' ll need from the store cupboard:

- Salt and pepper
- ½ cup water

Instructions:

1. In a food processor, place the lemon grass, green chilies, onions, ginger, coriander, basil, ground cumin, fish sauce, and lemon zest. Pulse until a smooth paste is formed. Set aside.
2. Heat the oil in a deep pan over medium flame and sauté the green paste made earlier. Stir for 30 seconds to a minute.
3. Stir in the chicken breasts and season with salt and pepper to taste. Cook for 5 minutes.
4. Pour in the coconut milk and water and bring to a boil. Once boiled, stir in the sweet peppers and baby corn. Continue cooking for another 5 minutes.

Nutrition Facts Per Serving:

Calories 195, Total Fat 9.4g, Saturated Fat 4.6g, Total Carbs 15.1g, Net Carbs g, Protein 9.4g, Sugar: 1.5g, Fiber: 1.9g, Sodium: 129mg, Potassium: 309mg

Indian Spice Chicken Curry

Ingredients:

- 1 tablespoon olive oil
- 1 lb. chicken breast, diced
- 1 teaspoon cayenne pepper
- ½ teaspoon cumin
- 5 potatoes, peeled and diced
- 1 can coconut milk

What you'll need from the store cupboard:

- Salt to taste

Instructions:

1. Heat oil in a pan over medium flame.
2. Stir in the chicken and season with salt to taste. Cook for 5 minutes while stirring constantly.
3. Stir in the cayenne pepper and cumin. Toast for 30 seconds.
4. Add in the potatoes and coconut milk. Season with more salt and pepper to taste.
5. Bring to boil and allow to cook the chicken for another 10 minutes.

Nutrition Facts Per Serving:

Calories 592, Total Fat 14.5g, Saturated Fat 3.7g, Total Carbs 82.8g, Net Carbs 71.9g, Protein 33.4g, Sugar: 4.9g, Fiber: 10.9g, Sodium: 153mg, Potassium: 2334 mg

Maple Peanut Sesame Chicken

Prep time: 8 hours, **Cook time:** 30 minutes; **Serves:** 4

Ingredients:

- 1-pound chicken tenders, bones and skin removed
- 2 tablespoons natural and sugar-free peanut butter
- 1 tablespoon sesame oil
- 3 tablespoons reduced sodium tamari
- 1 teaspoon ground ginger
- 1 ½ tablespoons pure maple syrup
- 1 tablespoon sesame seeds

What you'll need from the store cupboard:

- None

Instructions:

1. Place all ingredients except for the sesame seeds in a Ziploc bag and allow the chicken to marinate in the fridge for at least 8 hours.
2. Heat the oven to 350^0F.
3. Place the chicken in a baking dish and bake in the oven for 30 minutes.
4. Meanwhile, pour the marinade in a saucepan and heat for 10 minutes or until the sauce thickens.
5. Halfway through the cooking time, brush the chicken with the thickened marinade. Put the chicken back in the oven and continue cooking.
6. Toss in the sesame seeds before serving.

Nutrition Facts Per Serving:

Calories 307, Total Fat 16.8g, Saturated Fat 2.8g, Total Carbs 11.4g, Net Carbs 9.8g, Protein 28.7g, Sugar: 6.5g, Fiber:1.6g, Sodium: 160mg, Potassium: 449mg

Coconut Chicken Strips

Prep time: 10 minutes, Cook time: 15 minutes; Serves: 4

Ingredients:

- 1 lb. skinless and boneless chicken breasts, sliced into thick pieces
- ¾ cup shredded coconut
- 1 teaspoon dried basil
- 1 egg, beaten

What you' ll need from the store cupboard:

- Salt and pepper

Instructions:

1. Preheat the oven to 400⁰F.
2. Line a baking pan with parchment paper.
3. Pat dry the chicken strips and set aside.
4. In a bowl, combine the shredded coconut and basil. Season with salt and pepper. In another bowl, place the beaten egg.
5. Dip the chicken strips in egg first then in the coconut mixture.
6. Arrange on the baking pan or tray.
7. Bake for 15 minutes.

Nutrition Facts Per Serving:

Calories 177, Total Fat 5.5g, Saturated Fat 1.3g, Total Carbs 2.1g, Net Carbs 1.5g, Protein 28.1g, Sugar: 1.3g, Fiber: 0.6g, Sodium: 124mg, Potassium: 535mg

Balsamic Marinated Grilled Chicken

Ingredients:

- 4 chicken cutlets
- ¼ cup balsamic vinegar
- 2 tablespoons Dijon mustard
- 1 teaspoon dried rosemary of your choice
- 2 tablespoons olive oil

What you' ll need from the store cupboard:

- salt and pepper to taste

Instructions:

1. Place all ingredients in a Ziploc bag and shake well to coat the chicken with the other ingredients. Allow to marinate inside the fridge for at least 2 hours.
2. Preheat the grill to medium and place the chicken on the hot grill.
3. Cover the grill and cook the chicken for 8 minutes on each side.

Nutrition Facts Per Serving:

Calories 578, Total Fat 33.9g, Saturated Fat 8.7g, Total Carbs 3.4g, Net Carbs g, Protein 60.9g, Sugar: 2.4g, Fiber: 0.4g, Sodium: 272mg, Potassium: 671mg

Chicken Tikka Masala

Ingredients:

- 1 tablespoon ground cumin
- 1 tablespoon paprika
- 2 teaspoons garam masala
- 1 teaspoon ground chili pepper
- 1 teaspoon ground turmeric
- 1 teaspoon ground coriander
- ½ teaspoon asofatedia (optional)
- 1 ½ cups lactose-free yoghurt
- 2 tablespoon ginger root, minced
- 1 tablespoon oil
- 1 cup thinly sliced green scallions
- 2 cups chipped fennel bulb
- 2 cups chopped rutabaga
- 1 ½ pounds boneless chicken breasts
- 1 can crushed tomato

What you' ll need from the store cupboard:

- Salt and pepper to taste

Instructions:

1. In a small bowl, mix the cumin, paprika, garam masala, chili pepper, turmeric, coriander, and asofatedia. Season with salt and pepper to taste.
2. Divide the spice mixture in half. Combine one half with a third of the yogurt and the other half with ginger.
3. Cut the chicken breasts into thick strips and place in a large Ziploc bag. Pour the yoghurt and spice mixture and marinate for 3 hours inside the fridge.
4. Heat oil over medium flame and allow the chicken to brown at 3 minutes on each side.
5. Place the chicken in a foil-lined baking tray and cook in a broiler for 15 minutes.
6. Meanwhile, using the same skillet, stir in green scallions, fennel, and rutabaga. Stir for 1 minute or until wilted. Add the crushed tomatoes. Cook for another 10 minutes or until the vegetables are cooked.
7. Serve the chicken tikka with the sauce

Nutrition Facts Per Serving:

Calories 257, Total Fat 8.2g, Saturated Fat 2.6g, Total Carbs 17.8g, Net Carbs 12.9g, Protein 28.7g, Sugar: 11.1g, Fiber: 4.9g, Sodium: 150mg, Potassium: 1038mg

Chapter 8 Low FODMAP Vegetable Recipes

Roasted Vegetables with Rosemary and Feta

Prep time: 10 minutes, **Cook time:** 30 minutes; **Serves:** 4

Ingredients:

- 1 zucchini, chopped
- 1 red bell pepper, seeded and chopped
- 1 yellow bell pepper, seeded and chopped
- 2 carrots, peeled and chopped
- 2 tablespoons olive oil
- 1 tablespoon dried rosemary
- ½ cup feta cheese

What you' ll need from the store cupboard:

- Salt and pepper to taste

Instructions:

1. Preheat the oven to 350^0F and line a baking tray with parchment paper.
2. Place all vegetables in a baking tray and drizzle with olive oil. Season with rosemary, salt and pepper to taste.
3. Bake in the oven for 30 minutes. Make sure to give the baking tray a shake every 10 minutes for even cooking.
4. Once the vegetables are cooked, put on a serving plate and add feta.
5. Serve.

Nutrition Facts Per Serving:

Calories 135, Total Fat 11g, Saturated Fat 3.8g, Total Carbs 6.8g, Net Carbs 5.4g, Protein 3.6g, Sugar: 2.2g, Fiber: 1.4g, Sodium: 188mg, Potassium: 216mg

Ratatouille Casserole

Ingredients:

- 5 tablespoons olive oil
- 1 eggplant, sliced
- 1 zucchini, sliced
- 1 red bell pepper, seeded and sliced
- 1 can diced tomatoes
- 2 tablespoons chopped thyme
- 2 tablespoons chopped oregano
- 2 tablespoons chopped rosemary
- ½ cup white wine
- 3 basil leaves, torn
- 4 parsley leaves, torn
- 1 cup grated Parmigiano cheese
- 2 cups Gruyere cheese

What you' ll need from the store cupboard:

- Salt and pepper to taste

Instructions:

1. Preheat the oven to 375⁰F and spray a casserole dish with oil.
2. Heat the oil in a skillet and wilt the eggplants, zucchini, and red bell pepper. Season with salt and pepper to taste.
3. Place the vegetables on a casserole dish.
4. In a bowl, combine the tomatoes, thyme, oregano, rosemary, and white wine.
5. Pour over the vegetables and top with basil and parsley. Top with Parmigiano cheese and Gruyere cheese.
6. Bake in the oven for 20 minutes.

Nutrition Facts Per Serving:

Calories 298, Total Fat 24.6g, Saturated Fat 10.6g, Total Carbs 6.1g, Net Carbs 3.3g, Protein 15g, Sugar: 3.7g, Fiber: 2.8g, Sodium: 365mg, Potassium: 287mg

Vegetable Shepherd's Pie

Prep time: 10 minutes, Cook time: 30 minutes; Serves: 4

Ingredients:

- 1 lb. potatoes, peeled and diced
- 3 tablespoons nutritional yeast
- 1 tablespoon oil
- 1 cup leeks (green part only), chopped
- 3 large carrots, peeled and finely diced
- 1 wedge (6-ounce) kabocha squash, peeled and finely diced
- 1 can lentils, drained and rinsed thoroughly
- 1 can tomatoes, crushed
- ¼ cup pumpkin seeds
- ¼ teaspoon paprika
- ½ teaspoon dried thyme

What you' ll need from the store cupboard:

- Salt and pepper to taste

Instructions:

1. Preheat the oven to 375⁰F and grease a large baking dish.
2. Place potatoes in a pot and pour in enough water. Bring to a boil until the potatoes are soft. Drain the potatoes and put in a bowl. Add in the nutritional yeast and mash. Set aside.
3. In a large skillet, heat the oil over medium flame. Sauté the green leeks for 30 seconds until fragrant. Stir in the carrots, squash lentils, tomatoes, and pumpkin seeds. Add in the paprika and thyme. Season with salt and pepper to taste. Cover the skillet with lid and allow the vegetables to cook for 5 minutes.
4. Place the vegetables in a baking dish and spread evenly. Spread the potatoes on top of the vegetables.
5. Place in the oven and bake for 15 minutes.

Nutrition Facts Per Serving:

Calories 234, Total Fat 7.6g, Saturated Fat 1.2g, Total Carbs 34.9g, Net Carbs g, Protein 9.4g, Sugar: 6.5g, Fiber: 6.7g, Sodium: 470mg, Potassium: 1420mg

Winter Roasted Vegetable Salad

Prep time: 5 minutes, **Cook time:** 15 minutes; **Serves:** 2

Ingredients:

- 2 cups broccoli, cut into florets
- 2 cups yellow potatoes, scrubbed and halved
- 2 cups green beans
- 1 ½ teaspoon extra virgin olive oil
- 1 cup lettuce leaves
- 1 cup green onions, green part only
- 1 cup cooked quinoa
- ¼ cup red wine
- ¼ cup extra virgin olive oil
- 2 teaspoons Dijon mustard

What you'll need from the store cupboard:

- Salt and pepper to taste

Instructions:

1. Preheat the oven to 400^0F.
2. Line a baking tray with parchment paper.
3. In a bowl, toss together the broccoli, potatoes, beans, and olive oil. Season with salt and pepper to taste.
4. Place seasoned vegetable in a baking tray.
5. Roast in the oven for 15 minutes. Make sure to toss the vegetables every 5 minutes for even cooking.
6. Place the roasted vegetables in a salad bowl and add in the lettuce, green onions and cooked quinoa.
7. Make the salad dressing by combining the red wine, olive oil, and mustard. Season with salt and pepper to taste.
8. Drizzle the dressing onto the salad.
9. Toss to coat.

Nutrition Facts Per Serving:

Calories 408, Total Fat 16.3g, Saturated Fat 2.2g, Total Carbs 56.8g, Net Carbs 45.8g, Protein 11.1g, Sugar: 5.1g, Fiber: 11g, Sodium: 357mg, Potassium: 1167mg

Cobb Salad

Ingredients:

- 1 bag mixed salad greens, rinsed and chopped
- 2 big Roma tomatoes, diced
- 4 slices bacon, fried and crumbled
- 2 cups cooked chicken, shredded
- 4 hard-boiled eggs, diced
- ½ cup Kalamata olives, pitted and halved
- ¼ cup minced chives
- 2 tablespoons red wine vinegar
- 2 teaspoons Dijon mustard
- 1 teaspoon maple syrup
- ¼ cup olive oil

What you' ll need from the store cupboard:

- Salt and pepper to taste

Instructions:

1. Place the salad greens, tomatoes, bacon, chicken, boiled eggs, olives, and chives in a bowl.
2. In another bowl, mix together the red wine vinegar, Dijon mustard, maple syrup, and olive oil Season with olive oil.
3. Drizzle the salad with the dressing and toss to coat.

Nutrition Facts Per Serving:

Calories 645, Total Fat 58.1g, Saturated Fat 11g, Total Carbs 5.4g, Net Carbs 3.4g, Protein 24.6g, Sugar: 0.2g, Fiber: 2g, Sodium: 436mg, Potassium: 834mg

Low FODMAP Lentil Dal

Ingredients:

- 2 tablespoons olive oil
- 2 Roma tomatoes, diced
- 1 tablespoon ginger, finely chopped
- 1 teaspoon ground turmeric
- ¾ teaspoon garam masala
- ½ teaspoon ground cumin
- ½ teaspoon ground coriander
- ½ jalapeno pepper, sliced in half
- 1 can lentils, rinsed thoroughly and drained
- ½ cup canned coconut milk
- Juice from 1 lime

What you'll need from the store cupboard:

- Salt to taste

Instructions:

1. Heat the oil in a saucepan over medium flame.
2. Sauté the tomatoes, ginger, turmeric, garam masala, cumin, and coriander. Keep stirring for 1 minute or until the tomatoes have wilted.
3. Stir in the jalapeno pepper and lentils. Stir for another minute before adding in the coconut milk.
4. Season with salt to taste and the juice from 1 lime.
5. Bring to a boil and cook for 10 minutes.

Nutrition Facts Per Serving:

Calories 148, Total Fat 14.1g, Saturated Fat 7.3g, Total Carbs 5.9g, Net Carbs g, Protein 1.44g, Sugar: 2.9g, Fiber: 1.7g, Sodium: 9mg, Potassium: 269mg

Fruit and Walnut Salad

Prep time: 5 minutes, **Cook time:** 0 minutes; **Serves:** 1

Ingredients:

- 1 cup lettuce, torn
- 20 blueberries
- 1 tablespoon feta cheese, crumbled
- 10 walnut halves

What you'll need from the store cupboard:

- None

Instructions:

1. Dry the lettuce and place on a serving plate.
2. Crumble the feta cheese over the lettuce leaves and add fruits and nuts.

Nutrition Facts Per Serving:

Calories 198, Total Fat 16.5g, Saturated Fat 3.3g, Total Carbs 9.2g, Net Carbs g, Protein 6.5g, Sugar: 4.9g, Fiber: 2.6g, Sodium: 252mg, Potassium: 277mg

Asian-Inspired Quinoa Salad

Prep time: 10 minutes, Cook time: 0 minutes; Serves: 4

Ingredients:

- 1 cup quinoa, cooked in 1 ½ cups of water
- 1 large red bell pepper, seeded and diced
- 2 medium Lebanese cucumbers, diced
- 1 large carrot, peeled and grated
- ½ cup fresh mint, chopped
- ½ cup coriander, chopped
- Juice from 2 lemons
- 1 ½ tablespoons fish sauce
- 2 teaspoons minced ginger
- 2 teaspoons sesame oil
- A dash of cayenne pepper

What you'll need from the store cupboard:

- Salt and pepper to taste

Instructions:

1. Place in a salad bowl the quinoa, red bell pepper, cucumber, carrots, mint, and coriander.
2. In another bowl, mix together the lemon juice, fish sauce, ginger, oil, and cayenne pepper. Season with salt and pepper to taste.
3. Drizzle the dressing over the salad and toss to coat.

Nutrition Facts Per Serving:

Calories 153, Total Fat 6g, Saturated Fat 1.5g, Total Carbs 17.8g, Net Carbs 14.7g, Protein 8.7g, Sugar: 4.7g, Fiber: 3.1g, Sodium: 775mg, Potassium: 472mg

Low FODMAP Potato Salad

Prep time: 5 minutes, Cook time: 10 minutes; Serves: 2

Ingredients:

- 4 medium potatoes, scrubbed
- 5 slices of bacon
- 2 drops balsamic vinegar
- 2 drops olive oil
- Fresh mint for garnish, chopped

What you'll need from the store cupboard:

- Salt and pepper to taste

Instructions:

1. Boil the potatoes in a pot for 10 minutes or until soft. Drain and peel.
2. Meanwhile, fry the bacon for 3 minutes on each side or until crispy. Crumble.
3. Slice the potatoes and place in a bowl. Season with balsamic vinegar, olive oil, salt and pepper to taste.
4. Garnish with mint last.

Nutrition Facts Per Serving:

Calories 833, Total Fat 26.2g, Saturated Fat 0.1g, Total Carbs 74.9g, Net Carbs 65.6g, Protein 16.7g, Sugar: 3.8g, Fiber: 9.4g, Sodium: 331mg, Potassium: 674mg

Beef Bourguignon

Prep time: 10 minutes, **Cook time:** 6 hours; **Serves:** 4

Ingredients:

- ¼ cup tapioca flour
- 1 teaspoon cumin powder
- 18 oz chuck steak, sliced into strips
- 2 tablespoons olive oil
- 2 cups dry red wine
- 1 tablespoon tomato paste
- 2 carrots, peeled and chopped
- 2 zucchinis, chopped
- 1 bay leaf
- 1 teaspoon dried rosemary

What you' ll need from the store cupboard:

- Salt and pepper to taste

Instructions:

1. In a bowl, mix together the flour, salt, pepper, and cumin powder.
2. Toss in the beef slices into the flour mixture.
3. Heat the olive oil in a large skillet over medium flame and sauté the beef slices until brown. Continue cooking for 6 minutes and remove the meat from the pan.
4. Using the same pan, add wine to the pan and scrape the beef residue while heating.
5. Place the contents in the pan on a slow cooker and add in the rest of the ingredients including the beef.
6. Close the slow cooker and cook for 6 hours on low.

Nutrition Facts Per Serving:

Calories 314, Total Fat 15.2g, Saturated Fat 4.5g, Total Carbs 11.8g, Net Carbs 10.7g, Protein 27.8g, Sugar: 1.6g, Fiber: 1.1g, Sodium: 120mg, Potassium: 723mg

Steak and Potatoes Sheet Pan Meal

Prep time: 10 minutes, **Cook time:** 30 minutes; **Serves:** 4

Ingredients:

- 1 ½ lbs. baby potatoes, quartered
- 1 red bell pepper, seeded and cubed
- 1 green bell pepper, seeded and cubed
- 1 ½ lb. top sirloin steak, cut into thick strips

What you'll need from the store cupboard:

- Salt and pepper to taste

Instructions:

1. Preheat the oven to 400⁰F and line a baking sheet with aluminum foil.
2. In a bowl, mix the potatoes, peppers, steak, and olive oil. Season with salt and pepper to taste.
3. Bake for 30 minutes until the steaks and potatoes are done.

Nutrition Facts Per Serving:

Calories 461, Total Fat 19.2g, Saturated Fat 7.6g, Total Carbs 31.8g, Net Carbs 27.1, Protein 39.1g, Sugar: 2.5g, Fiber: 4.1g, Sodium: 102mg, Potassium: 1337mg

French Oven Beef

Prep time: 5 minutes, **Cook time:** 3 hours; **Serves:** 4

Ingredients:

- 1 lb. beef chuck, sliced
- 1 cup fennel bulb, diced
- 1 medium celery stalk, diced
- 6 medium carrots,
- 4 medium parsnips
- 4 medium potatoes
- ¼ cup tapioca starch
- 1 cup tomato juice
- 1 tablespoon maple syrup

What you' ll need from the store cupboard:

- Salt and pepper to taste

Instructions:

1. Preheat the oven to 300^0F.
2. Place all ingredients in a heat-proof deep dish and mix until well combined.
3. Bake the dish for 3 hours on medium heat.

Nutrition Facts Per Serving:

Calories 548, Total Fat 7.3g, Saturated Fat 2.1g, Total Carbs 91.2g, Net Carbs g, Protein 32.8g, Sugar: 14.4g, Fiber: 13.8g, Sodium: 288mg, Potassium: 2671mg

Beef Stroganoff

Prep time: 5 minutes, Cook time: 20 minutes; Serves: 4

Ingredients:

- 2 teaspoons olive oil
- 1 cup white cabbage, thinly sliced
- 1 ½ cups green tops of spring onions, thinly sliced
- 1 can sliced champignon mushrooms, drained and rinsed well
- ½ lb. beef strips
- 1 tablespoon tapioca flour
- 1 teaspoon sweet paprika
- 2 tablespoon tomato paste
- 2 teaspoon Dijon mustard
- 2 tablespoons coconut yoghurt

What you'll need from the store cupboard:

- 1 ¼ cups water
- Salt and pepper to taste

Instructions:

1. Heat oil in a large pan on medium flame. Stir in the cabbages and cook for 4 minutes or until wilted. Add the green onions and sliced mushrooms. Cook for another 2 minutes while stirring constantly. Set aside.
2. Using the same pan, increase the heat to medium high and stir in the beef strips and cook until brown.
3. While the beef strips are cooking, mix together the tapioca starch and paprika. Add the flour mixture into the beef and reduce the heat to medium. Stir until the beef strips are coated. Cook for another minute while stirring constantly.
4. Add in the tomato paste, Dijon mustard, and water. Season with salt and pepper to taste.
5. Close the lid and allow to boil. Once boiling, lower the heat and add in the cabbage and mushroom mixture.
6. Allow to simmer for 10 minutes before adding the coconut yoghurt last.

Nutrition Facts Per Serving:

Calories 122, Total Fat 4.2g, Saturated Fat 0.8g, Total Carbs 8.2g, Net Carbs 6.4g, Protein 14.3g, Sugar: 3.4g, Fiber: 1.8g, Sodium: 82mg, Potassium: 413mg

Lamb Casserole

Prep time: 10 minutes, **Cook time:** 2 hours and 10 minutes; **Serves:** 4

Ingredients:

- 1 tablespoon coconut oil
- 2 lbs. lamb meat, cut into chunks
- 1 tablespoon coriander
- 1 teaspoon ground cardamom
- 1 tablespoon ground cumin
- ½ cup red wine
- ½ cup tomato paste
- 1 can of lentils, rinsed and drained thoroughly
- 3 large carrots, chopped

What you'll need from the store cupboard:

- Salt and pepper to taste
- 2 cups water

Instructions:

1. In a large pan, heat the oil over medium flame.
2. Cook the lamb while stirring constantly until all sides turn brown.
3. Add the coriander, cardamom, and cumin. Season with salt and pepper to taste.
4. Stir in the red wine, tomato paste, lentils, and carrots. Pour in water and bring to a boil.
5. Cook the lamb for 2 hours on medium meat or until the meat is tender.

Nutrition Facts Per Serving:

Calories 407, Total Fat 15.4g, Saturated Fat 7.4g, Total Carbs 16.7g, Net Carbs 13.5g, Protein 48.9g, Sugar: 6.6g, Fiber: 3.2g, Sodium: 221mg, Potassium: 1263mg

Lamb Skewers with Oregano

Prep time: 10 minutes, **Cook time:** 12 minutes; **Serves:** 4

Ingredients:

- 2 pounds lamb, cut into small chunks
- 3 teaspoons dried oregano
- 2 teaspoons sweet paprika
- 2 teaspoon extra virgin olive oil

What you' ll need from the store cupboard:

- Salt and pepper to taste

Instructions:

1. Thread the lamb chunks through 8 skewers. Set aside on a plate.
2. In a bowl, combine the rest of the ingredients and mix well. Season with salt and pepper to taste.
3. Brush the skewered lamb meat with the spice mixture.
4. Heat the grill to medium and cook for 6 minutes on each side.

Nutrition Facts Per Serving:

Calories 595, Total Fat 39.3g, Saturated Fat 18.2g, Total Carbs 1.1g, Net Carbs 0.4g, Protein 55.9g, Sugar: 0.2g, Fiber: 0.7g, Sodium: 192mg, Potassium: 719mg

Slow Cooked Roasted Lamb with Potatoes

Prep time: 5 minutes, **Cook time:** 10 hours; **Serves:** 8

Ingredients:

- 10 medium sized potatoes, peeled and halved
- 2 pounds leg of lamb, whole bone-in
- 2 sprigs fresh thyme
- 2 sprigs fresh rosemary
- 1 cup red wine
- 1 bay leaf

What you'll need from the store cupboard:

- Salt and pepper to taste

Instructions:

1. Place the potatoes in the slow cooker. Put the lamb leg on top.
2. Add in the rest of the ingredients and season with salt and pepper to taste.
3. Close the lid and cook for 8 to 10 hours on low.

Nutrition Facts Per Serving:

Calories 509, Total Fat 6.4g, Saturated Fat 2.3g, Total Carbs 80.9g, Net Carbs g, Protein 32.4g, Sugar: 3.9g, Fiber: 10.1g, Sodium: 103mg, Potassium: 2289mg

Easy Lamb Curry

Prep time: 10 minutes, **Cook time:** 50 minutes; **Serves:** 8

Ingredients:

- 1 tablespoon olive oil
- 1 tablespoon grated fresh ginger
- ½ cup chopped leeks, green parts only
- ½ cup chopped scallions, green parts only
- 2 teaspoons curry powder
- ½ teaspoon garam masala
- ½ teaspoon turmeric
- ¼ teaspoon cayenne pepper
- 1 lb. lamb meat, cut into cubes
- 1 can diced tomatoes
- 1 bay leaf
- ½ cup coconut yoghurt

What you'll need from the store cupboard:

- Salt and pepper to taste
- ½ cup water

Instructions:

1. Heat the oil in a large skillet over medium flame.
2. Sauté the ginger, leeks, and scallions until fragrant.
3. Stir in the curry powder, garam masala, turmeric, and cayenne pepper. Allow to toast for a minute.
4. Add in the lamb meat and continue stirring. Season with salt and pepper to taste. Cook for 5 minutes until the herbs have infused into the lamb meat.
5. Stir in the tomatoes and bay leaf. Pour in water.
6. Bring to a boil and cook for 45 minutes or until the lamb meat is tender.
7. Stir in the coconut yoghurt last.

Nutrition Facts Per Serving:

Calories 107, Total Fat 4.8g, Saturated Fat 1.4g, Total Carbs 4g, Net Carbs 2.9g, Protein 12.1g, Sugar: 1.4g, Fiber: 1.1g, Sodium: 85mg, Potassium: 288mg

Lamb and Spinach Curry

Prep time: 10 minutes, **Cook time:** 50 minutes; **Serves:** 4

Ingredients:

- 2 tablespoons olive oil
- 1-inch ginger, grated
- 2 red chilies, seeded and chopped
- 2 teaspoons ground cumin
- 2 teaspoons ground coriander
- 1 teaspoon turmeric
- 1 lb. lamb meat, diced
- 1 can crushed tomatoes
- 1 cup spinach
- 5 green tops of spring onion, chopped
- A handful of fresh coriander leaves

What you'll need from the store cupboard:

- Salt and pepper to taste
- Water

Instructions:

1. Heat the oil in a large pan over medium flame and sauté the ginger and red chilies for 30 seconds.
2. Stir in the cumin, coriander, and turmeric and toast for another 30 seconds.
3. Add in the lamb meat and continue stirring until all sides of the meat turn golden. Season with salt and pepper to taste.
4. Add in the tomatoes and pour enough water to submerge the meat.
5. Close the lid and bring to a boil. Cook for 45 minutes or until the meat is tender.
6. Once the meat is cooked, add in the spinach, spring onions, and coriander leaves.

Nutrition Facts Per Serving:

Calories 257, Total Fat 13.2g, Saturated Fat 3.3g, Total Carbs 10.1g, Net Carbs 7.1g, Protein 24.8g, Sugar: 4.8g, Fiber: 3g, Sodium: 155mg, Potassium: 664mg

Short Rib Beef Stew

Prep time: 10 minutes, **Cook time:** 1 hour and 10 minutes; **Serves:** 8

Ingredients:

- 2 bone-in beef ribs, cut into chunks
- 3 tablespoons olive oil
- 1 lb. rutabaga, peeled and cut into 2-inch pieces
- 2 lb. carrots, peeled and cut into 2-inch pieces
- 1 teaspoon dried thyme
- 1 tablespoon tapioca flour
- 2 tablespoon butter, melted
- 1 cup fresh parsley

What you' ll need from the store cupboard:

- Salt and pepper to taste
- 5 cups water

Instructions:

1. Season the meat with salt and pepper to taste. Set aside.
2. Heat oil in a pot over medium flame and stir in the seasoned meat. Continue stirring until all sides of the meat turn golden brown.
3. Place the rutabaga, carrots, and thyme into the pot. Add in water and bring to a boil.
4. Cook for 60 minutes until the beef is tender.
5. Meanwhile, mix the tapioca flour and butter until a smooth paste is formed.
6. Once the beef is soft, stir in the butter paste and continue stirring until the sauce thickens.
7. Garnish with parsley last.

Nutrition Facts Per Serving:

Calories 1008, Total Fat 69.8g, Saturated Fat 25.7g, Total Carbs 18.1g, Net Carbs g, Protein 78.9g, Sugar: 8.1g, Fiber: 4.8g, Sodium: 343mg, Potassium: 1610mg

Moroccan Beef Stew

Prep time: 10 minutes, **Cook time:** 60 minutes; **Serves:** 10

Ingredients:

- 3 pounds beef chuck roasts, sliced thickly
- 4 teaspoons olive oil
- 1 teaspoon ginger
- 1 teaspoon ground cumin
- 1 teaspoon ground turmeric
- 1 teaspoon ground cinnamon
- 2 medium carrots, peeled and cut into large chunks
- 1 medium parsnips, peeled and cut into large chunks
- 1 can diced tomatoes
- 1 lb. sweet potatoes, peeled and cubed
- 1 cup leek leaves, chopped finely

What you' ll need from the store cupboard:

- Salt and pepper to taste
- 1 cup water
- 2 tablespoons brown sugar

Instructions:

1. Season the meat with salt and pepper to taste.
2. Heat oil in a large pan or skillet over medium heat and stir in the ginger and seasoned beef. Keep stirring until the beef turns golden.
3. Stir in the cumin, turmeric, and cinnamon until the beef and stir for another 30 seconds.
4. Add in the carrots, parsnips, tomatoes, and sweet potatoes. Add in water and brown sugar. Season with more salt and pepper if desired.
5. Close the lid and bring to a boil. Cook for 50 minutes or until the beef is tender.
6. Add in the leeks last before serving.

Nutrition Facts Per Serving:

Calories 316, Total Fat 13.5g, Saturated Fat 4.9g, Total Carbs 11.6g, Net Carbs 9.5g, Protein 37.7g, Sugar: 1.8g, Fiber: 2.1g, Sodium: 144mg, Potassium: 762mg

Minted Lamb Casserole

Prep time: 10 minutes, Cook time: 65 minutes; Serves: 4

Ingredients:

- 1 tablespoon olive oil
- 1 lb. lamb meat, cut into chunks
- 3 carrots, peeled and chopped
- 4 parsnips, peeled and chopped
- 3 potatoes, peeled and chopped
- 1 can crushed tomato
- ½ cup white wine
- 1 cup mint leaves, chopped

What you' ll need from the store cupboard:

- Salt and pepper to taste

Instructions:

1. Preheat the oven for 375^0F.
2. Heat oil in a skillet over medium flame and brown the lamb meat on all sides for about 5 minutes. Set aside.
3. Put the carrots, parsnips, and potatoes in a casserole dish and put in the lamb on top. Pour tomatoes on top and white wine. Season with salt and pepper to taste.
4. Put the mint leaves on top.
5. Bake in the oven for 60 minutes or until the lamb is soft.

Nutrition Facts Per Serving:

Calories 539, Total Fat 10g, Saturated Fat 2.8g, Total Carbs 82.8g, Net Carbs 68.9g, Protein 32.1g, Sugar: 12.6g, Fiber: 13.9g, Sodium: 189mg, Potassium: 2322mg

Chapter 10 Low FODMAP Pasta, Noodle, And Rice Recipes

Salmon and Spinach

Prep time: 10 minutes, **Cook time:** 20 minutes; **Serves:** 4

Ingredients:

- 1 package gluten-free spaghetti noodles
- 1 tablespoon olive oil
- 1 ½ cup fresh spinach
- 1 can canned sliced mushrooms
- 2 cups lactose-free cream cheese
- 1 cup smoked salmon flakes
- Juice from 1 lemon

What you' ll need from the store cupboard:

- Water
- Salt and pepper to taste

Instructions:

1. Place water in a deep pot and bring to a boil. Cook spaghetti noodles according to package instructions. Drain the noodles and set aside once cooked.
2. Heat olive oil in a pan over medium heat and wilt the spinach and set aside.
3. Using the same pan, stir in the mushrooms. Add in the cream cheese and pour water. Season with salt and pepper to taste. Bring to a boil and add in the salmon flakes.
4. Stir in the spaghetti noodles. Add the wilted spinach.
5. Drizzle with lemon juice before serving.

Nutrition Facts Per Serving:

Calories 406, Total Fat 5.9 g, Saturated Fat 1.5g, Total Carbs 59.3g, Net Carbs 51g, Protein 32.5g, Sugar: 9.7g, Fiber: 8.3g, Sodium: 125mg, Potassium: 558mg

Spaghetti Bolognese

Prep time: 10 minutes, Cook time: 20 minutes; Serves: 5

Ingredients:

- 1 package gluten-free spaghetti noodles
- 1 tablespoon olive oil
- ½ lb. minced beef
- 1 cup green leeks, chopped
- 1 can crushed tomatoes
- 2 teaspoons Italian herbs
- 2 large carrots, grated
- 1 ½ cups chopped green beans
- 4 cups baby spinach, chopped
- 1 cup parmesan cheese
- A handful of basil, torn

What you' ll need from the store cupboard:

- Salt and pepper to taste

Instructions:

1. Cook the spaghetti noodles according to package instructions. Once cooked, drain the noodles and set aside.
2. Heat the olive oil over medium heat. Stir in the beef and leeks and cook for 3 minutes while stirring constantly.
3. Add in the tomatoes, herbs, carrots, and green beans. Season with salt and pepper to taste and adjust the moisture by adding more water if needed.
4. Allow to simmer for 10 minutes until the vegetables are soft.
5. Stir in the spinach and cooked noodles last.
6. Garnish with parmesan and basil leaves.

Nutrition Facts Per Serving:

Calories 388, Total Fat 12.2g, Saturated Fat 4.4g, Total Carbs 49.9g, Net Carbs 40.2g, Protein 24.9g, Sugar: 4.6g, Fiber: 9.7g, Sodium: 491mg, Potassium: 652mg

Pad Thai With Shrimps

Prep time: 10 minutes, **Cook time:** 6 minutes; Serves: 4

Ingredients:

- 1 package rice noodle
- 2 tablespoons olive oil
- 1 lb. large shrimps, peeled and deveined
- 1 red bell pepper, thinly sliced
- ¼ cup fish sauce
- ¼ cup white sugar
- 2 tablespoons rice vinegar
- 1 tablespoons ground paprika
- 2 teaspoons low sodium tamari
- 1 large egg, fried and cut into strips
- 2 green onions, green parts only chopped
- 1 cup fresh bean sprouts
- 1 teaspoon sesame seeds
- Freshly chopped cilantro leaves

What you' ll need from the store cupboard:

- Salt to taste

Instructions:

1. Cook the rice noodles according to package instructions. Drain and set aside.
2. Heat the olive oil in pan over medium heat and stir in the shrimps and bell pepper. Season with salt to taste and cook for 4 minutes until the shrimps turn red. Set aside.
3. In a mixing bowl, combine the fish sauce, white sugar, rice vinegar, and paprika. Add in the tamari.
4. Assemble the Pad Thai. Place the noodles at the bottom of the bowl and place the shrimps and bell pepper on top. Add egg strips, green onions, and bean sprouts. Drizzle with the sauce.
5. Garnish with sesame seeds and cilantro seeds.

Nutrition Facts Per Serving:

Calories 429, Total Fat 13.5g, Saturated Fat 2g, Total Carbs 52.7g, Net Carbs 48.5g, Protein 24.4g, Sugar: 4.7g, Fiber: 4.2g, Sodium: 215mg, Potassium: 423mg

Coconut Chicken Rice Noodle

Ingredients:

- 1 package rice noodle
- 2 tablespoons coconut oil
- 1 lb. chicken breasts
- 1 zucchini, sliced
- 1 bell pepper, seeded and sliced
- 2 carrots, peeled and sliced
- 1 can coconut milk

What you' ll need from the store cupboard:

- Salt and pepper to taste

Instructions:

1. Cook the rice noodles according to package instructions. Drain and set aside.
2. Heat coconut oil in a deep pan over medium heat and fry the chicken breasts for 3 minutes on each side or until they turn golden brown.
3. Stir in the zucchini, bell pepper, and carrots. Season with salt and pepper to taste. Stir for 1 minute.
4. Add in the coconut milk.
5. Cover the pan with lid and simmer for 6 minutes.
6. Add cooked noodles last.

Nutrition Facts Per Serving:

Calories 415, Total Fat 13.9g, Saturated Fat 7.1g, Total Carbs 22.5g, Net Carbs 19.1g, Protein 19.6g, Sugar: 1.2g, Fiber: 3.4g, Sodium: 102mg, Potassium: 347mg

Beef and Vegetable Stir Fry with Oyster Sauce

Ingredients:

- 2 tablespoons sesame oil
- ½ lb. beef slices
- ½ carrot, peeled and julienned
- ½ cup broccoli florets
- ½ cup chopped bok choy
- 6 oz rice noodles
- 2 tablespoons oyster sauce
- 1 teaspoon lime juice

What you'll need from the store cupboard:

- Salt and pepper to taste
- Water

Instructions:

1. Heat the sesame oil in pan over medium flame and stir in the beef slices. Season with salt and pepper to taste. Cook for 3 minutes.
2. Stir in the vegetables and rice noodles. Pour in a few tablespoons of water to adjust the moisture. Season with oyster sauce.
3. Keep stirring until the noodles and vegetables are cooked.
4. Drizzle with lime juice last.

Nutrition Facts Per Serving:

Calories 611, Total Fat 49.5g, Saturated Fat 16.4g, Total Carbs 11.7g, Net Carbs 10.7g, Protein 29.7g, Sugar: 5.3g, Fiber: 1g, Sodium: 638mg, Potassium: 503mg

Chicken and Rice

Prep time: 5 minutes, **Cook time:** 35 minutes; **Serves:** 4

Ingredients:

- 4 skinless boneless chicken breasts, around 1 ½ lbs.
- 1 ¾ teaspoon ground cumin
- 1 ¾ teaspoon paprika powder
- 1 tablespoon coconut oil
- 1 red and green bell peppers, seeded and chopped
- 1 large tomato, chopped
- 1 tablespoon ginger, chopped
- 1 teaspoon turmeric powder
- 1 cup white rice, uncooked

What you' ll need from the store cupboard:

- Salt and pepper to taste
- 2 cups water

Instructions:

1. Season the chicken breasts with cumin, paprika, salt, and pepper.
2. Heat oil in a pan over medium flame and stir in the seasoned chicken breasts. Allow to brown on all sides for at least 3 to 4 minutes. Set aside.
3. Using the same pan, stir in the green bell peppers, tomatoes, ginger, and turmeric. Allow the vegetables to sweat.
4. Add the rice and season with salt and pepper to taste. Pour in water.
5. Put lid on the pan and cook the rice for 30 minutes on low heat.
6. Halfway through the cooking time, place the chicken on top of the rice and continue cooking.

Nutrition Facts Per Serving:

Calories 545, Total Fat 11.2g, Saturated Fat 4.6g, Total Carbs 41.3g, Net Carbs 38.8g, Protein 65.2g, Sugar: 1.4g, Fiber: 2.5g, Sodium: 131mg, Potassium: 1113mg

Tuna Fried Rice

Prep time: 10 minutes, **Cook time:** 33 minutes; **Serves:** 4

Ingredients:

- ¼ tablespoon sesame oil
- ¼ tablespoon grated ginger
- 2 tablespoons green onions, green parts chopped
- 1/3 red bell pepper, seeded and sliced
- 1/3 carrot, peeled and grated
- 1 can tuna in brine, drained
- 1/3 cup long grain white rice
- ½ teaspoon Thai fish sauce
- ½ tablespoons soy sauce
- 2 tablespoons coriander leaves, chopped

What you' ll need from the store cupboard:

- Salt to taste
- ½ teaspoon white sugar

Instructions:

1. Heat sesame oil in pan over medium flame. Sauté the ginger and green onions until fragrant.
2. Stir in the rest of the ingredients. Pour water to adjust the mixture. Give a good mix before covering the pan.
3. Cook on low for 30 minutes or until the rice is cooked through.

Nutrition Facts Per Serving:

Calories 131, Total Fat 3.4g, Saturated Fat 0.9g, Total Carbs 13.7g, Net Carbs 13.2g, Protein 11.1g, Sugar: 0.9g, Fiber:0.5g, Sodium: 218mg, Potassium: 437mg.

Tuna Noodle Casserole

Prep time: 10 minutes, Cook time: 20 minutes; Serves: 4

Ingredients:

- 1 package 7 ounces gluten-free pasta
- ¼ cup unsalted butter
- ½ cup green part of the leek, chopped
- ½ cup green scallions, green part chopped
- 3 ½ ounces oyster mushrooms
- ¼ cup peas
- ¼ cup tapioca starch
- ¾ cup coconut milk
- 2 teaspoons soy sauce
- 2 ounces mozzarella cheese

What you' ll need from the store cupboard:

- Salt and pepper to taste

Instructions:

1. Preheat the oven to 350^0F. Grease the casserole dish with non-stick spray.
2. Cook the pasta in a large pot with boiling water and cook according to package instructions. Drain and set aside.
3. Melt the butter over medium heat in a skillet and sauté the leeks and scallion for 30 seconds. Stir in the oyster mushrooms and peas and cook for 2 minutes.
4. Stir in the tapioca starch and coconut milk. Allow to simmer and season with soy sauce, salt and pepper to taste.
5. Place the cooked pasta in the casserole dish and pour in the sauce.
6. Top with cheese.
7. Bake in the oven for 15 minutes.

Nutrition Facts Per Serving:

Calories 262, Total Fat 19.1g, Saturated Fat 14.4g, Total Carbs 17.7g, Net Carbs 15g, Protein 7.5g, Sugar: 3.3g, Fiber: 2.7g, Sodium: 205mg, Potassium 290 mg

Chapter 11 Low FODMAP Dessert Recipes

Bread Pudding with Blueberries

Prep time: 10 minutes, **Cook time:** 40 minutes; **Serves:** 2

Ingredients:

- 1 extra-large egg
- 2/3 cup unsweetened almond milk
- 1 tablespoon maple syrup
- ¼ teaspoon vanilla extract
- 4 slices of gluten-free bread
- ½ cup blueberries
- A dash of ground cinnamon

What you'll need from the store cupboard:

- None

Instructions:

1. Preheat the oven to 375^0F.
2. In a bowl, whisk the eggs, almond milk, and maple syrup until well combined. Add in the vanilla extract.
3. Cut the crusts from the bread and slice the bread into tiny cubes. Place the bread cubes in a greased baking dish and pour the egg mixture. Top with blueberries and sprinkle with a dash of cinnamon.
4. Bake for 40 minutes or until the egg mixture is set and the top has browned and puffed up.

Nutrition Facts Per Serving:

Calories 268, Total Fat 6.5g, Saturated Fat 2.6g, Total Carbs 44.9g, Net Carbs 42.8g, Protein 7.8g, Sugar: 25.6g, Fiber: 2.1g, Sodium: 238mg, Potassium: 215mg

Millet Chocolate Pudding

Prep time: 10 minutes, Cook time: 0 minutes; Serves: 4

Ingredients:

- 1 lb. cooked millet
- 2 cup unsweetened almond milk
- ½ medium banana
- ¼ cup cocoa powder
- 2 tablespoons maple syrup

What you' ll need from the store cupboard:

- None

Instructions:

1. Pour all ingredients in a blender and pulse until smooth.
2. Pour the chocolate mixture into bowls and allow to set in the fridge before serving.

Nutrition Facts Per Serving:

Calories 260, Total Fat 5.8g, Saturated Fat 2.9g, Total Carbs 45.9g, Net Carbs 42.4g, Protein 8.9g, Sugar: 14.3g, Fiber: 3.5g, Sodium: 27mg, Potassium: 443mg

Chocolate Coconut Pudding

Ingredients:

- 2 cups coconut milk
- ¼ cup cocoa powder
- ¼ cup pure maple syrup
- 3 tablespoons arrowroot starch
- ½ cup almond milk
- 3 oz dark chocolate chips
- ¾ teaspoon vanilla extract
- 1 ½ tablespoons unsweetened shredded coconut

What you'll need from the store cupboard:

- 1/8 teaspoon sea salt

Instructions:

1. Pour the coconut milk in a saucepan and add salt, cocoa powder, and maple syrup. Heat the saucepan on low heat.
2. Meanwhile, mix together the arrow root starch and almond milk until the starch dissolves.
3. Once the coconut milk is warm, add the starch mixture and allow to boil until the milk thickens.
4. Turn off the heat and stir in the chocolate chips, vanilla extract, and coconut.
5. Place in ramekins and allow to set in the fridge overnight before serving.

Nutrition Facts Per Serving:

Calories 380, Total Fat 18.9g, Saturated Fat 10.6g, Total Carbs 47.2g, Net Carbs 41.7g, Protein 9.1g, Sugar: 34.8g, Fiber: 5.5g, Sodium: 117mg, Potassium: 719mg

Chocolate English Custard Recipes

Prep time: 10 minutes, **Cook time:** 10 minutes; **Serves:** 2

Ingredients:

- 1 ½ tablespoons tapioca starch
- 1 egg
- 1 tablespoon pure maple syrup
- ¾ cup almond milk
- 1 tablespoons water
- 1 ½ tablespoons cocoa powder

What you'll need from the store cupboard:

- None

Instructions:

1. Add all ingredients in a saucepan and whisk until all lumps are removed.
2. Place the saucepan on the stove and bring to a boil over low heat while stirring constantly.
3. Turn off the heat once the mixture thickens.
4. Pour into ramekins and refrigerate for 3 hours before serving.

Nutrition Facts Per Serving:

Calories 170, Total Fat 6.5g, Saturated Fat 2.1g, Total Carbs 24.6g, Net Carbs 21.4g, Protein 5.8g, Sugar: 16.2g, Fiber: 3.2g, Sodium: 340mg, Potassium: 892mg

Vanilla Maple Chia Pudding

Prep time: 10 minutes, Cook time: 0 minutes; Serves: 1

Ingredients:

- 3 tablespoons chia seeds
- 1 cup coconut milk
- ½ teaspoon vanilla extract
- 1 tablespoon maple syrup

What you'll need from the store cupboard:

- None

Instructions:

1. Mix all ingredients in a container and stir until well combined.
2. Place inside the fridge and allow to set overnight.

Nutrition Facts Per Serving:

Calories 280, Total Fat 12.6g, Saturated Fat 5.1g, Total Carbs 31.7g, Net Carbs 26.5g, Protein 10.2g, Sugar: 24.2g, Fiber: 5.2g, Sodium: 110mg, Potassium: 452mg

Dark Chocolate Gelato

Ingredients:

- 2 ¼ cups coconut milk
- ¾ cup lactose-free heavy cream
- 2 tablespoons arrow root starch
- ½ cup cocoa powder
- 4 oz dark chocolate

What you' ll need from the store cupboard:

- ¾ cup sugar

Instructions:

1. In a saucepan, place half of the coconut milk, cream, arrow root starch, cocoa powder, and dark chocolate. Add in the sugar.
2. Turn on the stove and bring the mixture to a simmer until it thickens. Turn off the heat and add the remaining milk. Mix until well combined.
3. Pour into an ice cream maker. Turn the ice cream maker for 3 hours until the mixture turns into a gelato.
4. If you don't have an ice cream maker, you can place the mixture in a lidded container. Place in the fridge for 8 hours but make sure that you mix the mixture every hour to create the creamy gelato texture.

Nutrition Facts Per Serving:

Calories 145, Total Fat 11.4g, Saturated Fat 9.1g, Total Carbs 11g, Net Carbs 7.5g, Protein 2.5g, Sugar: 3.4g, Fiber: 3.5g, Sodium: 20mg, Potassium: 299mg

Low FODMAP Rustic Carrot Cake

Prep time: 15 minutes, Cook time: 35 minutes; Serves: 24

Ingredients:

- 2 cups gluten-free all-purpose flour
- 2 teaspoons baking powder
- 1 teaspoon baking soda
- 1 cup vegetable oil
- 4 large eggs
- 2 teaspoons cinnamon
- 1 teaspoon vanilla extract
- 1-pound carrots, grated
- ¾ cup raisins

What you' ll need from the store cupboard:

- 1 teaspoon salt
- ¾ cup brown sugar

Instructions:

1. Preheat the oven to 350°F. Grease a cake pan or line with parchment paper.
2. In a bowl, whisk the flour, baking powder, baking soda, and salt. Pass through a sieve to aerate and remove lumps. Set aside.
3. In another bowl, combine the remaining ingredients. Mix until the sugar dissolves. This will be the wet ingredient.
4. Pour the wet ingredients over the dry ingredients and fold until combined.
5. Pour the batter into the prepared cake pan and bake for 35 minutes or until a toothpick inserted in the middle comes out clean.
6. Allow to cool down before removing from the cake pan.

Nutrition Facts Per Serving:

Calories 136, Total Fat 10g, Saturated Fat 1.8g, Total Carbs 10.1g, Net Carbs 9.2g, Protein 1.7g, Sugar: 0.9g, Fiber: 0.9g, Sodium: 15mg, Potassium: 76mg

Lemon Cake with Frosting

Prep time: 15 minutes, **Cook time:** 45 minutes; **Serves:** 10

Ingredients:

- 1 cup + 3 ½ tablespoons softened butter
- 2 cups gluten-free flour
- 4 tablespoons baking powder
- 4 eggs
- 4 tablespoons almond milk
- Zest from 1 lemon, grated
- 1 ½ cup powdered sugar
- 3 tablespoons lemon juice

What you' ll need from the store cupboard:

- 1 cup white sugar

Instructions:

1. Preheat the oven to 350⁰F. Grease a baking pan with butter.
2. In a large bowl, place 1 cup of the butter, flour, baking powder, eggs, almond milk, and lemon zest. Mix until well combined.
3. Pour the batter into the baking pan. Cover the pan with aluminum foil and bake for 45 minutes or until a toothpick inserted in the middle comes out clean.
4. Once cooked, allow the cake to cool.
5. While the cake is cooling, make the frosting by combining the remaining butter, powdered sugar, and lemon juice. Mix until well combined.
6. Once the cake is cooled, pour over the frosting.

Nutrition Facts Per Serving:

Calories 300, Total Fat 22.5g, Saturated Fat 12.8g, Total Carbs 20.9g, Net Carbs 20.7g, Protein 4.5g, Sugar: 15.6g, Fiber: 0.2g, Sodium: 227mg, Potassium: 98mg

Banana Cake

Ingredients:

- 4 oz softened butter
- 3 eggs
- 2 cups gluten-free flour
- 2 teaspoons baking powder
- 1 teaspoon cinnamon
- ½ cup yoghurt
- 1 cup mashed banana

What you' ll need from the store cupboard:

- ¼ cup brown sugar

Instructions:

1. Heat the oven to 350^0F and grease a baking dish with butter.
2. In a bowl, place the butter and sugar and mix with an electric blender until the mixture becomes fluffy and pale. Add eggs gradually and continue stirring.
3. Sift the flour, baking powder, and cinnamon into the butter mixture and add the yoghurt and banana. Stir until well combined.
4. Pour into the baking dish and bake for 45 minutes or until a toothpick inserted in the middle comes out clean.
5. Allow to cool before removing from the baking dish.

Nutrition Facts Per Serving:

Calories 231, Total Fat 16.1g, Saturated Fat 8.6g, Total Carbs 18.6g, Net Carbs 17g, Protein 5.1g, Sugar: 7.1g, Fiber: 1.6g, Sodium: 183mg, Potassium: 294mg

Butter Tarts

Prep time: minutes, Cook time: minutes; Serves: 24

Ingredients:

- 1 ½ cups gluten-free flour
- ¼ cup butter
- ¼ cup lard
- 1 egg yolk
- 1 teaspoon vinegar
- Iced water
- 1 egg
- 2 tablespoons butter, room temperature
- 1 teaspoon vanilla
- 1 teaspoon vinegar

What you'll need from the store cupboard:

- ¼ teaspoon salt
- ¾ cup brown sugar

Instructions:

1. Preheat the oven to 350^0F. Grease the tart mold with butter.
2. Make the tart crust first by whisking in together the gluten-free flour and add in the butter and lard in small batches until coarse crumb forms.
3. In a bowl, whisk together the egg yolk, vinegar, and a little bit of ice water until the mixture reaches ½ cup full. Gradually add the mixture into the crust and mix using your hands to create a pastry dough.
4. Press the dough into tart molds and allow to set inside the fridge for 2 hours.
5. Meanwhile, make the tart filing. Whisk the sugar, egg, butter, vanilla, and vinegar. Stir in the salt. Mix until well combined.
6. Pipe in the tart filling into prepared dough and bake in a 450^0F preheated oven for 30 minutes.
7. Allow to cool before removing from the tart mold.

Nutrition Facts Per Serving:

Calories 86, Total Fat 5.7g, Saturated Fat 2.8g, Total Carbs 8.4g, Net Carbs 8.3g, Protein 0.6g, Sugar: 6.8g, Fiber: 0.1g, Sodium: 65mg, Potassium: 23mg

Lime Cake

Ingredients:

- 2 ½ cups gluten-free flour
- 1 tablespoon baking powder
- 1 teaspoon xanthan gum
- 4 large eggs
- 1 cup canola oil
- 1 cup coconut milk
- 1 teaspoon vanilla extract
- 1 teaspoon lime extract

What you' ll need from the store cupboard:

- 2 cups sugar
- ½ teaspoon salt
- 1 tablespoon lime zest
- 3 tablespoons freshly squeezed lime juice

Instructions:

1. Preheat the oven to 350^0F and grease a cake pan with shortening or oil.
2. In a bowl, mix the flour, baking powder, and xanthan gum. Sift through a sieve to aerate the dry ingredients.
3. In another bowl, mix together the eggs, canola oil, coconut milk, vanilla extract, lime extract, sugar, salt, lime zest, and lime juice. Beat until the sugar dissolves and the liquid turns smooth.
4. Fold in the dry ingredients gradually and mix until the lumps are removed.
5. Pour the batter into the prepared pan. Tap the bottom of the pan to remove too much air within the batter.
6. Place in the oven and bake for 45 minutes.

Nutrition Facts Per Serving:

Calories 422, Total Fat 30.7g, Saturated Fat 3.4g, Total Carbs 35.2g, Net Carbs 34.9g, Protein 3.1g, Sugar: 26.5g, Fiber: 0.3g, Sodium: 221mg, Potassium: 114mg

Berry Crumb Cake

Ingredients:

- 2 cups gluten-free flour
- 1 teaspoon baking powder
- ¾ cup butter, cold
- ¾ cup coconut milk
- 1 tablespoon lemon juice
- 2 eggs
- 1 cup strawberries and blueberries

What you' ll need from the store cupboard:

- 1 cup sugar

Instructions:

1. Preheat the oven to 350^0F and lightly grease an 8x8 square pan.
2. In a bowl, add the sugar, baking powder, and sugar.
3. Add butter into the flour mixture gradually. Use a pastry blender until you achieve a crumb-like texture. Reserve half of the crumb mixture for the topping.
4. In another bowl, stir in the coconut milk, and lemon juice. Let it stand for 5 minutes.
5. Add into half of the flour mixture the eggs and milk and mix until well combined.
6. Fold in the berries.
7. Pour the mixture into the prepared pan and sprinkle on top the reserved crumb topping.
8. Bake for 50 minutes.
9. Allow to cool before slicing.

Nutrition Facts Per Serving:

Calories 171, Total Fat 12.7g, Saturated Fat 8.2g, Total Carbs 13.6g, Net Carbs 13g, Protein 1.9g, Sugar: 10.1g, Fiber: 0.6g, Sodium: 107mg, Potassium: 70mg

Chocolate Chunks Cookies

Ingredients:

- 2 1/3 cup gluten-free flour
- 1 teaspoon baking soda
- 1 cup unsalted butter, room temperature
- 1 cup light brown sugar
- 2 teaspoons vanilla extract
- 2 large eggs
- 12 oz dark chocolates, chopped
- 1 1/3 cups toasted pecan halves, chopped

What you' ll need from the store cupboard:

- 1 teaspoon salt

Instructions:

1. In a bowl, mix together the flour, baking soda, and salt. Sift the flour mixture to aerate. Set aside.
2. Place the butter in a bowl and add in the sugar and vanilla extract. Beat for 3 minutes until the mixture lightens. Add in the eggs one at a time.
3. Beat in the dry mixture until only a few streaks of flour remain.
4. Stir in the dark chocolates and pecans until well combined. Cover the bowl and chill for at least 4 hours.
5. Preheat the oven to 375^0F. Line a baking sheet with parchment paper. Position the rack in the upper thirds of the oven.
6. Form small balls from the dough and place on the baking sheet.
7. Bake for 15 minutes or until lightly brown.

Nutrition Facts Per Serving:

Calories 378, Total Fat 26.7g, Saturated Fat 12.3g, Total Carbs 32.2g, Net Carbs 28.5g, Protein 4.1g, Sugar: 21.7g, Fiber: 3.7g, Sodium: 47mg, Potassium: 262mg

Peanut Butter Oatmeal Chocolate Chip Cookies

Ingredients:

- 1 cup gluten-free flour
- ½ teaspoon xanthan gum
- 1 teaspoon baking soda
- 8 tablespoons unsalted butter, cold and cubed
- ½ cup natural creamy peanut butter
- 2/3 cup sugar
- 1 teaspoon pure vanilla extract
- 1 large egg
- ¾ cup gluten-free quick oats
- 1 cup semi-sweet mini chocolate chips

What you' ll need from the store cupboard:

- ¼ teaspoon salt

Instructions:

1. Preheat the oven to 350^0F. Line a baking sheet with parchment paper.
2. In a small bowl, mix together the gluten-free flour, xanthan gum, baking soda, and salt.
3. In another bowl, cream the butter and add in the peanut butter, sugar, and vanilla extract. Beat in the eggs and continue to beat until well-combined.
4. Gradually add the dry ingredients and mix until everything is incorporated.
5. Stir in the oats, chocolate chip cookies. Scoop the cookie dough and place on the cookie sheet.
6. Bake for 12 minutes.
7. Remove from the cookie sheet on the cooling rack before serving.

Nutrition Facts Per Serving:

Calories 199, Total Fat 10.3g, Saturated Fat 3.9g, Total Carbs 25.5g, Net Carbs 23.6, Protein 4.2g, Sugar: 15.8g, Fiber: 1.9g, Sodium: 65mg, Potassium: 161mg

Baked Peanut Butter Protein Bars

Prep time: 20 minutes, Cook time: 0 minutes; Serves: 12

Ingredients:

- 1 cup natural creamy peanut butter
- ¾ cup maple syrup
- 1 teaspoon vanilla bean paste
- 1 ½ cups gluten-free rolled oats
- 1 cup protein powder

What you' ll need from the store cupboard:

- None

Instructions:

1. Line a baking pan with parchment paper.
2. In a microwave-safe bowl, heat the peanut butter and maple syrup for 30 seconds. Stir then add in the vanilla bean paste then heat again for 30 seconds.
3. Stir in oats and protein powder.
4. Spread into the prepared pan and press using the back of the spoon.
5. Refrigerate for an hour and cut into 12 bars.

Nutrition Facts Per Serving:

Calories 271, Total Fat 14.9g, Saturated Fat 2.5g, Total Carbs 27.6g, Net Carbs 23.4g, Protein 14g, Sugar: 13.7g, Fiber: 4.2g, Sodium: 128mg, Potassium: 442mg

Gluten-Free Lemon Cookies

Prep time: 20 minutes, Cook time: 15 minutes; Serves: 20

Ingredients:

- ¼ cup coconut milk
- ¼ cup fresh lemon juice
- ½ cup butter
- 1 egg
- 1 teaspoon vanilla extract
- Zest of one lemon
- 1 teaspoon baking soda
- 1 teaspoon baking powder
- 2 ½ cups gluten-free flour
- ½ cup fresh lemon juice
- 2 cups powdered sugar

What you'll need from the store cupboard:

- 1 cup sugar

Instructions:

1. Preheat the oven to 350⁰F and grease a baking sheet with butter. Set aside.
2. Combine the milk and lemon juice in a bowl. Set aside.
3. Cream the butter and sugar using an electric mixer. Add in the egg and vanilla extract.
4. Add in the milk mixture to the butter mixture and fold. Set aside.
5. In another bowl, combine the lemon zest, baking powder, and flour.
6. Add the dry ingredients to the wet ingredients then fold.
7. Scoop cookie dough and place on the baking sheet. Press the dough using your fingers.
8. Bake for 15 minutes.
9. Allow the cookies to cool on a cooling rack.
10. Meanwhile, prepare the frosting by mixing the lemon juice and sugar.
11. Brush the top of the cookies with the frosting.

Nutrition Facts Per Serving:

Calories 110, Total Fat 5.9g, Saturated Fat 3.7g, Total Carbs 14.1g, Net Carbs 13.9g, Protein 0.9g, Sugar:10.3 g, Fiber: 0.2g, Sodium: 65mg, Potassium: 40mg

Granola Bars

Ingredients:

- 1 cup rice flake
- 1 cup millet flakes
- ½ cup dried cranberries
- ½ cup pumpkin seeds
- ¼ cup sunflower seeds
- ½ cup peanut butter
- 2 teaspoons malt syrup
- 1 teaspoon cinnamon powder

What you' ll need from the store cupboard:

- Coconut oil for greasing

Instructions:

1. Preheat the oven to 355°F and grease a small baking tray.
2. In a bowl, mix together the rice flakes, millet, cranberries, pumpkin seeds, and peanut butter.
3. In a blender, mix together the peanut butter, and malt syrup. Add in the cinnamon powder.
4. Pour into the granola mixture and mix well.
5. Press into the baking tray and bake for 15 minutes.
6. Allow to harden before cutting into bars.

Nutrition Facts Per Serving:

Calories 180, Total Fat 8.6g, Saturated Fat 1.4g, Total Carbs 23.4g, Net Carbs 19g, Protein 6.1g, Sugar: 4.4g, Fiber: 4.4g, Sodium: 175mg, Potassium: 270mg

CPSIA information can be obtained
at www.ICGtesting.com
Printed in the USA
LVHW101305040221
678375LV00005B/25

9 781637 330937